Doctors, nurses, patients, relatives, friends we were all doing our best to cope, to be hopeful, to do the right thing. But the bewilderment, shock and despair were there too, just below the surface. We knew what was happening but how could we understand why or how? They were ferocious times.

These images are beautiful, honest, intense and operatic. You can see the love there in black and white, picture after picture. And, as we know, love never dies.

Julian Clary, 2017

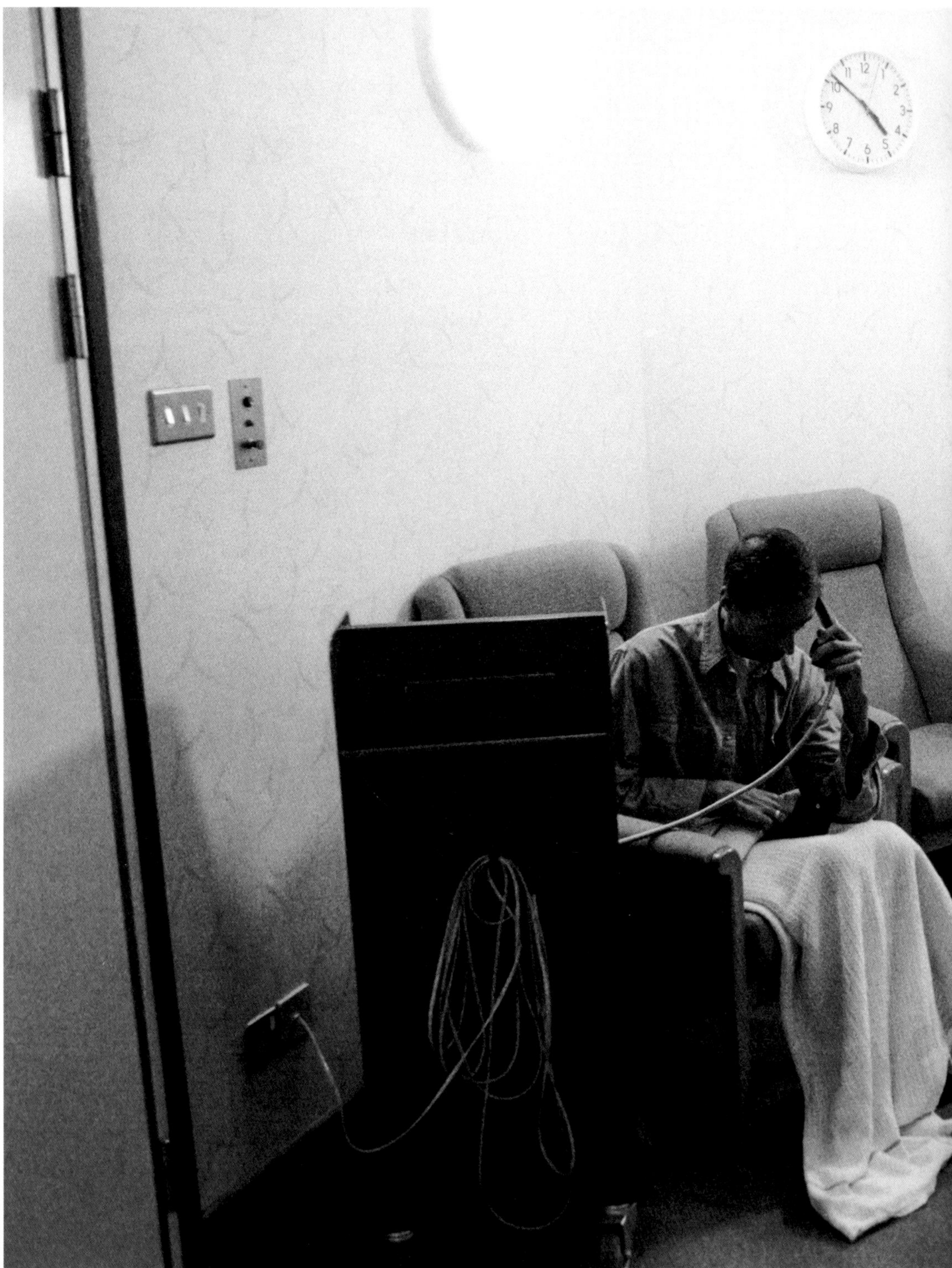

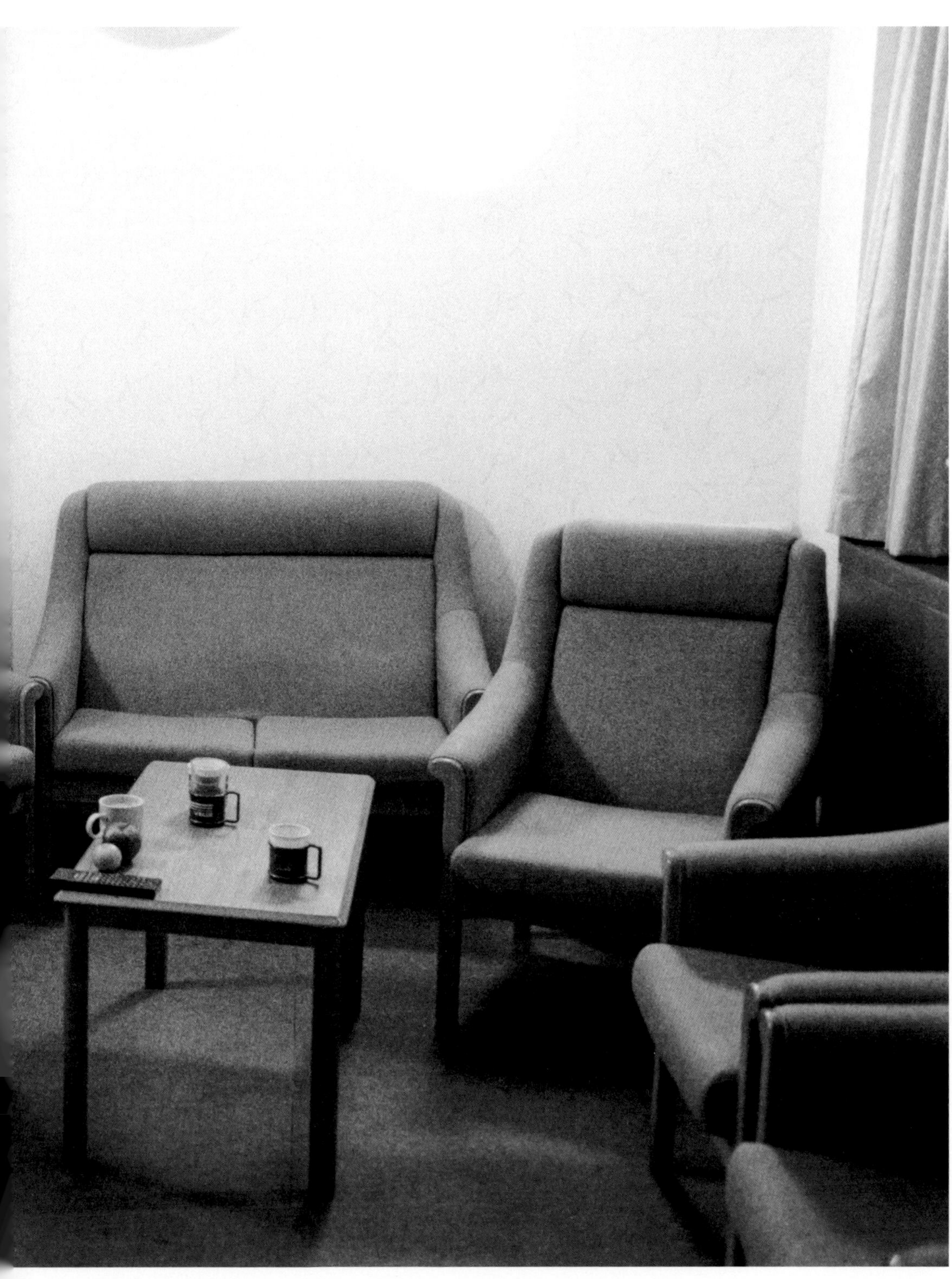

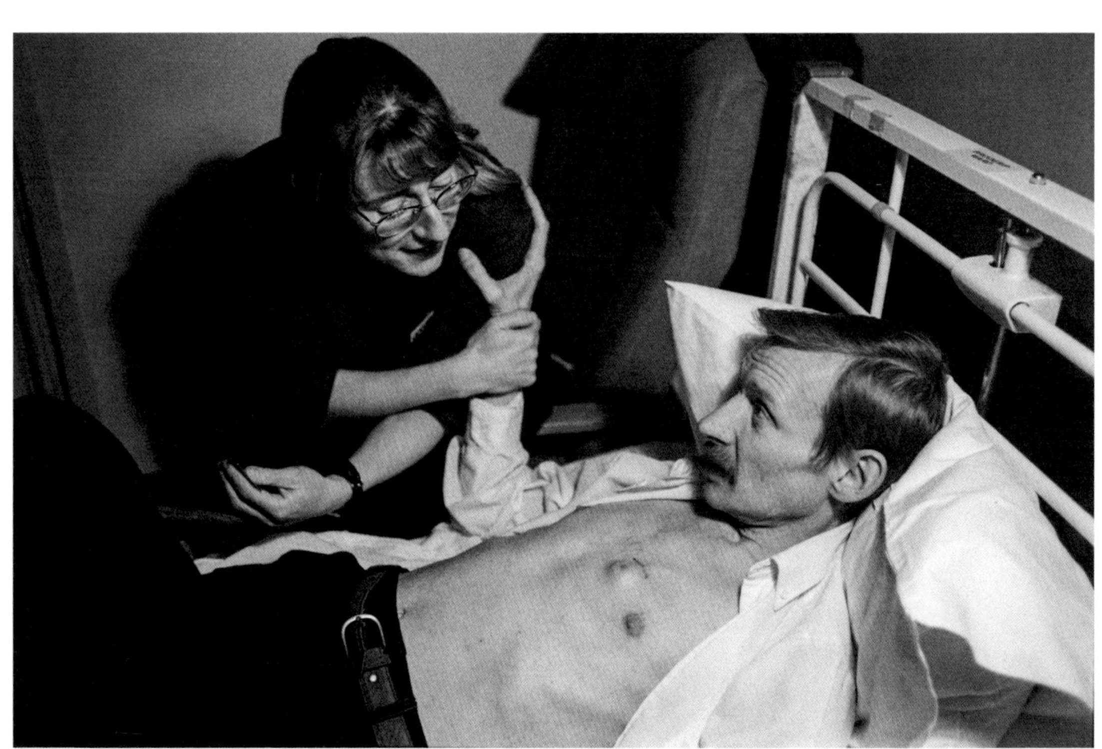

In 1993, I spent a number of weeks photographing the Broderip and Charles Bell wards in London's Middlesex Hospital as part of the Positive Lives project. This was the era before antiretroviral medications had become available, a very distinct and tragic time. All of the patients on the wards, many of whom were young, gay men, were facing the terrifying prospect of an early and painful death.

These were some of the few dedicated AIDS wards that existed in London, even more unusual for their decision to open themselves to being photographed. Considering the high levels of stigma and fear that existed at the time, the decision of these four patients to allow themselves, alongside their families, lovers and friends to be photographed was an act of considerable bravery.

During my time at the hospital, I photographed their treatment and many other aspects of ward life, including the intimate way in which the staff, patients and their families related to one another. Treatment was not a passive process, but rather an active engagement on the part of the patients, who were often extremely knowledgeable about their condition. The staff, too, became far more attached to their patients than was commonplace in hospitals at the time.

All of the patients in these photographs died soon after the pictures were taken. They were the unlucky ones, who became sick just before treatment became available. This was my first encounter with HIV/AIDS, one that greatly impacted the course of my life and subsequent photographic journey.

Coming back to these images now, twenty five years later, I am struck by how they now seem to have become part of history, marking a very particular moment in time and the evolution of medical and social responses to HIV. Going through my contact sheets I am reminded of the intensity of those moments, of the lives lived so brightly and the desperate sadness and loss for all those connected to John, Ian, Steven and Andre.

Gideon Mendel

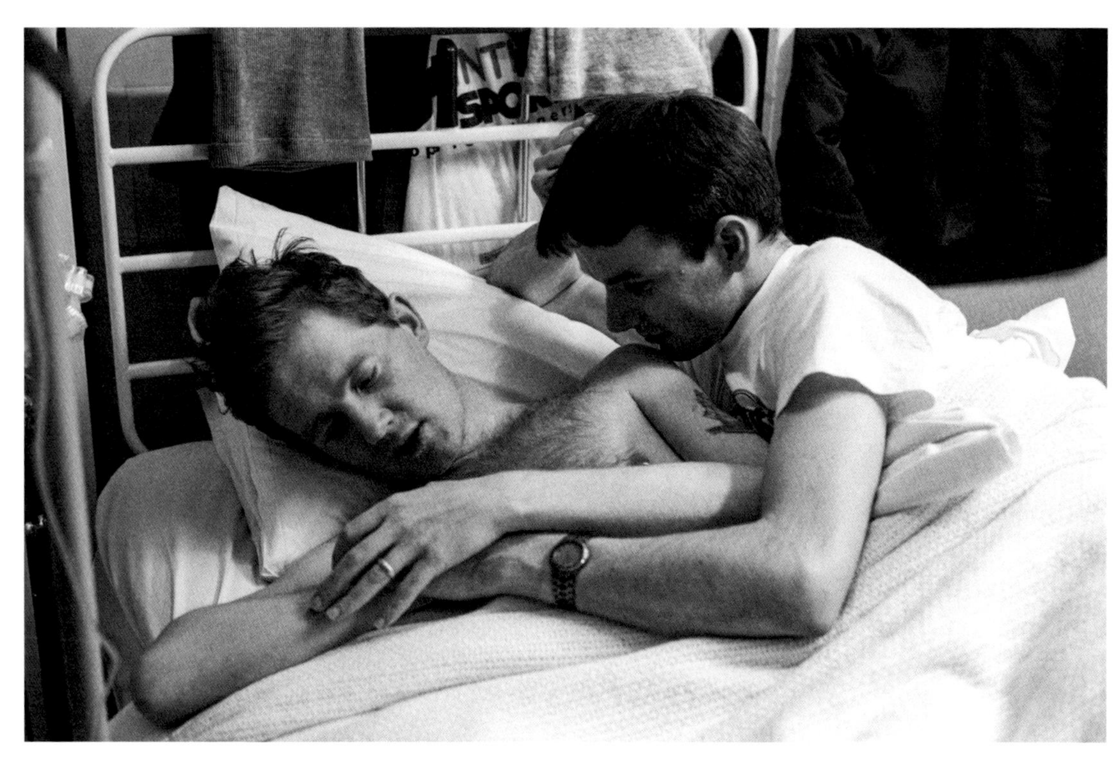

* * T R O L L E Y * *

The Ward
Gideon Mendel

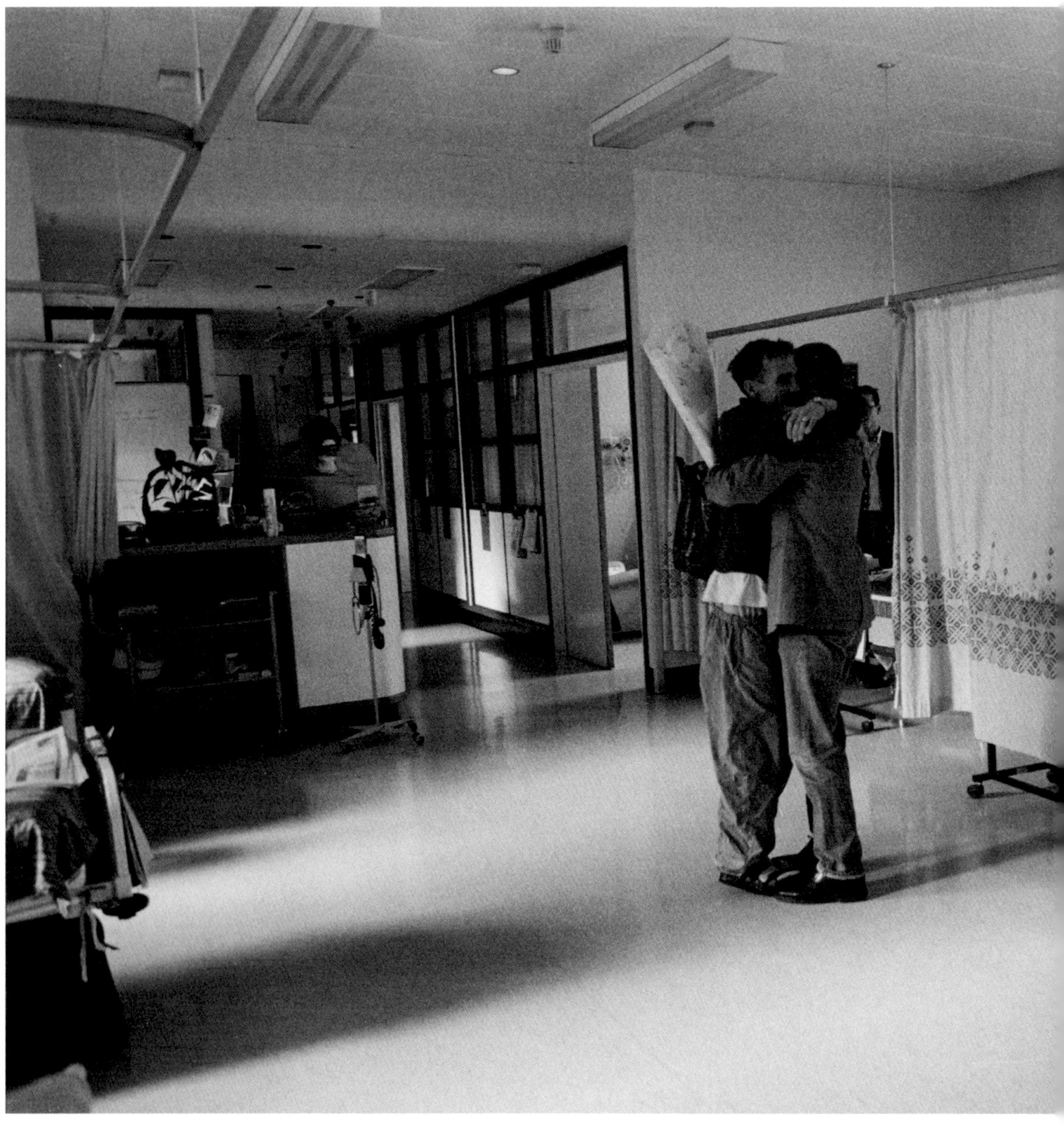

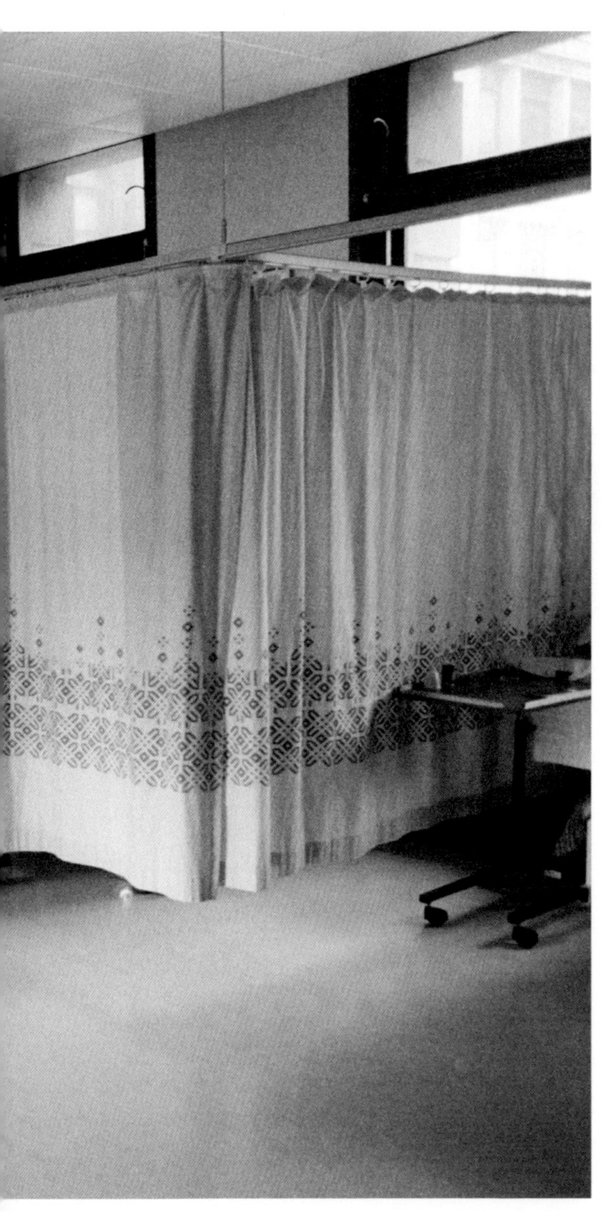

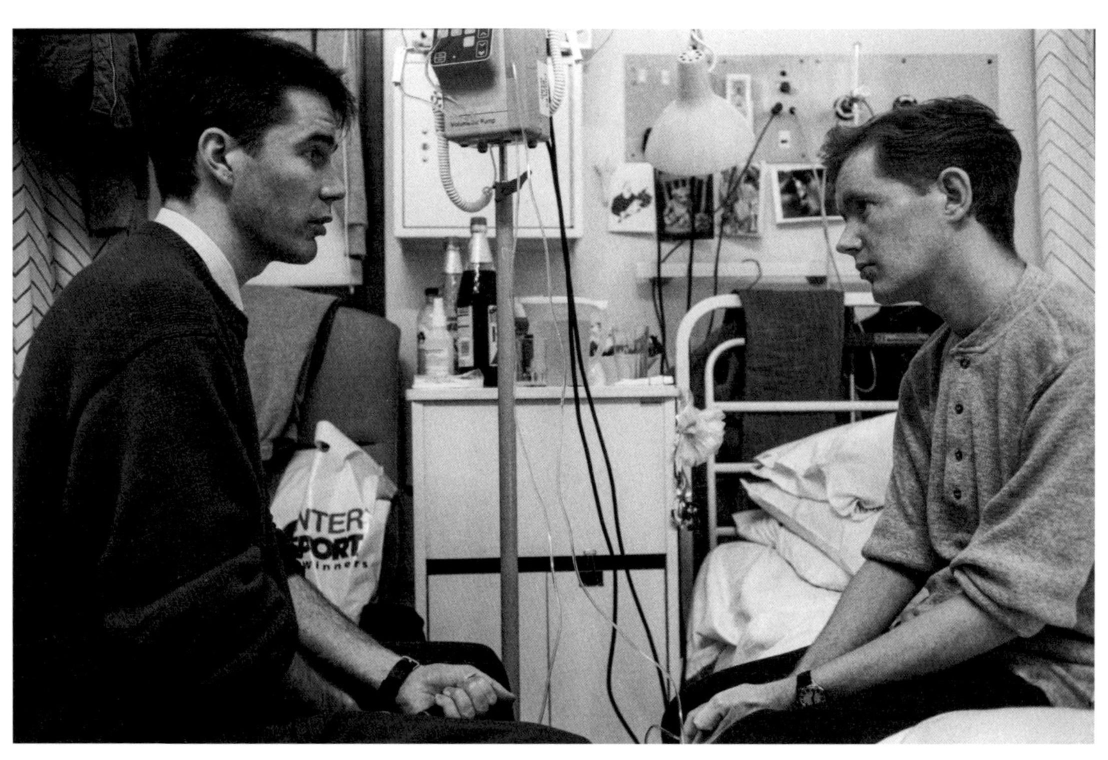

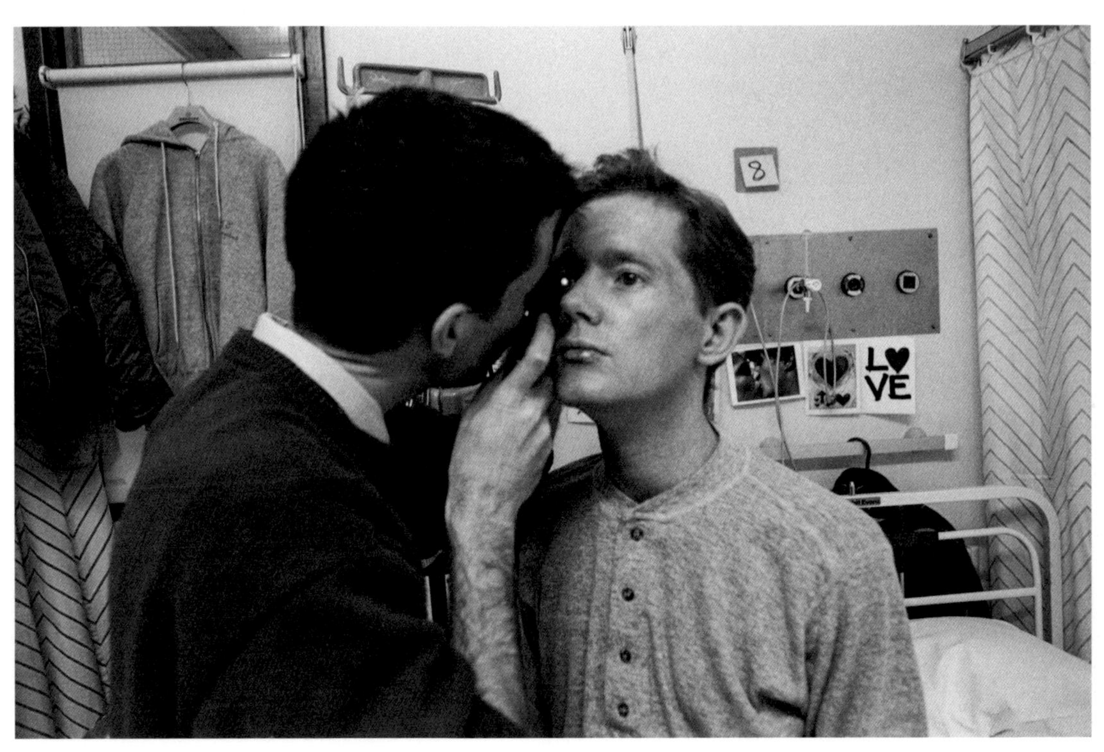

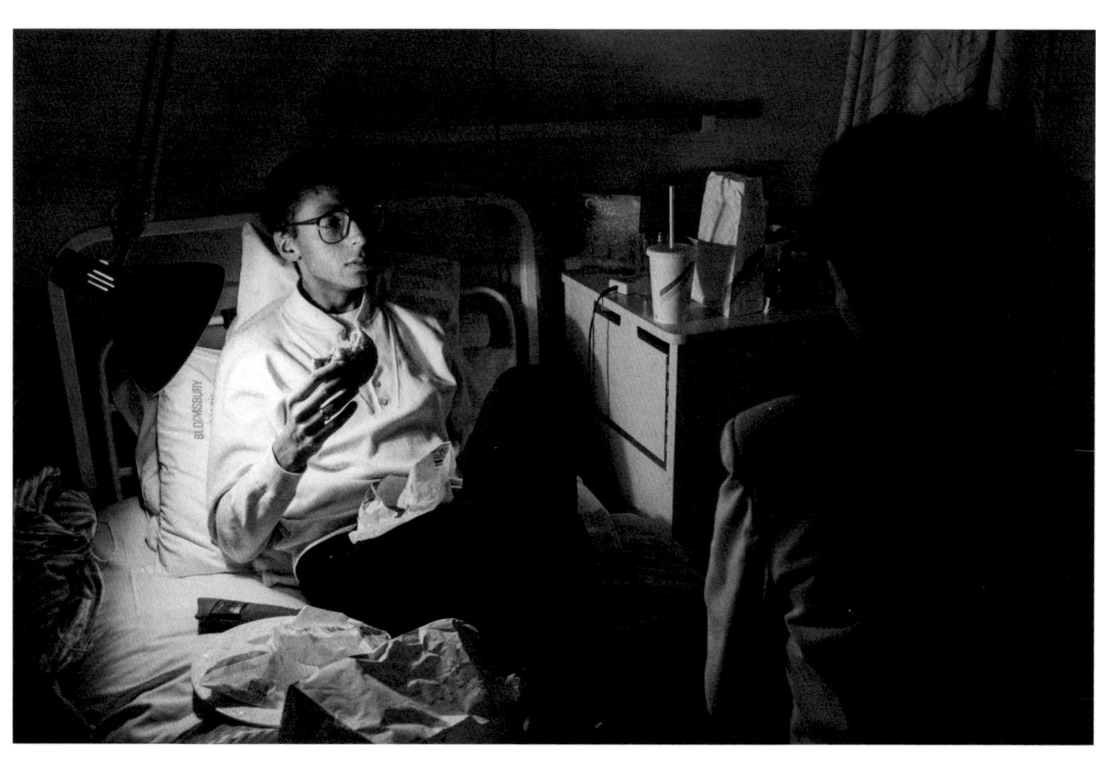

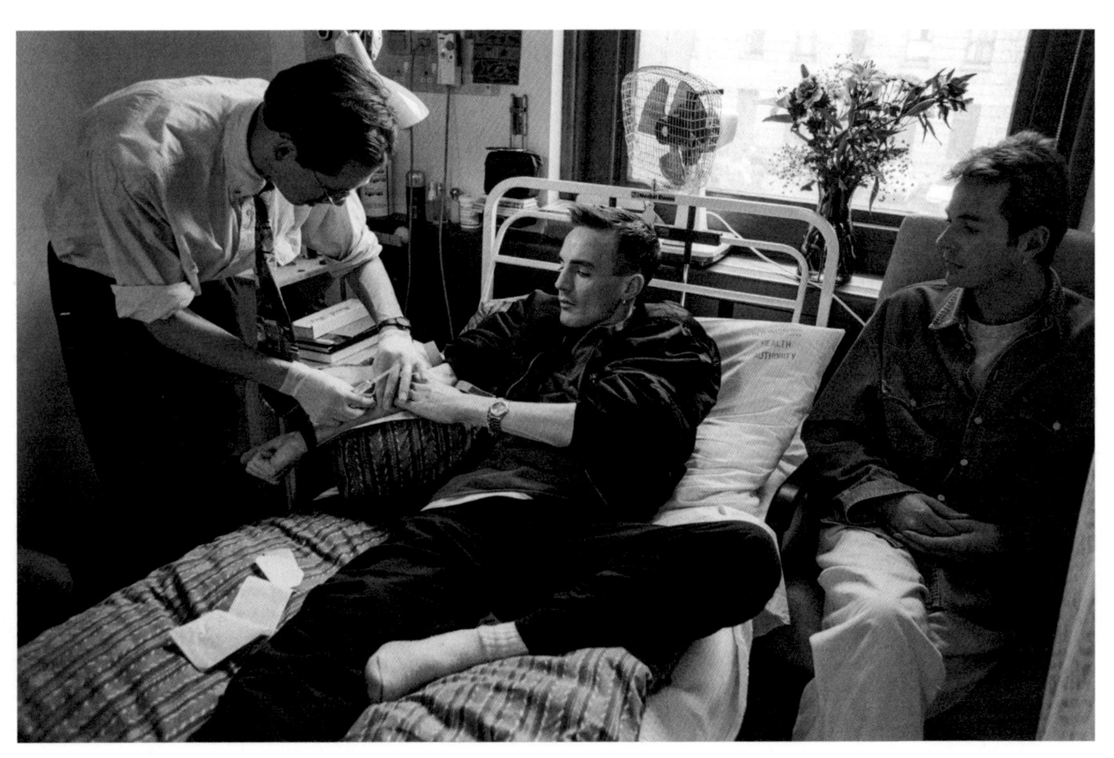

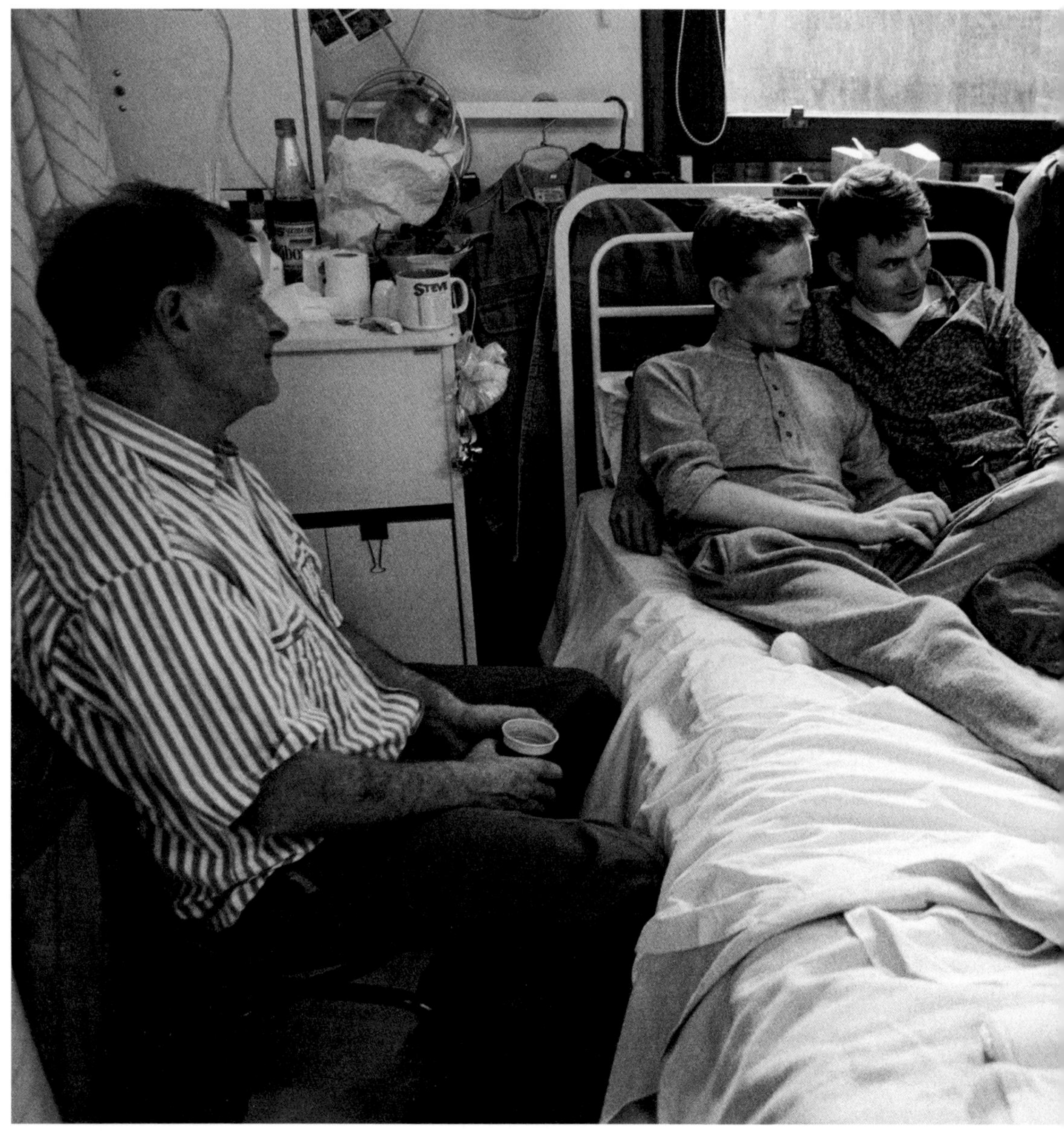

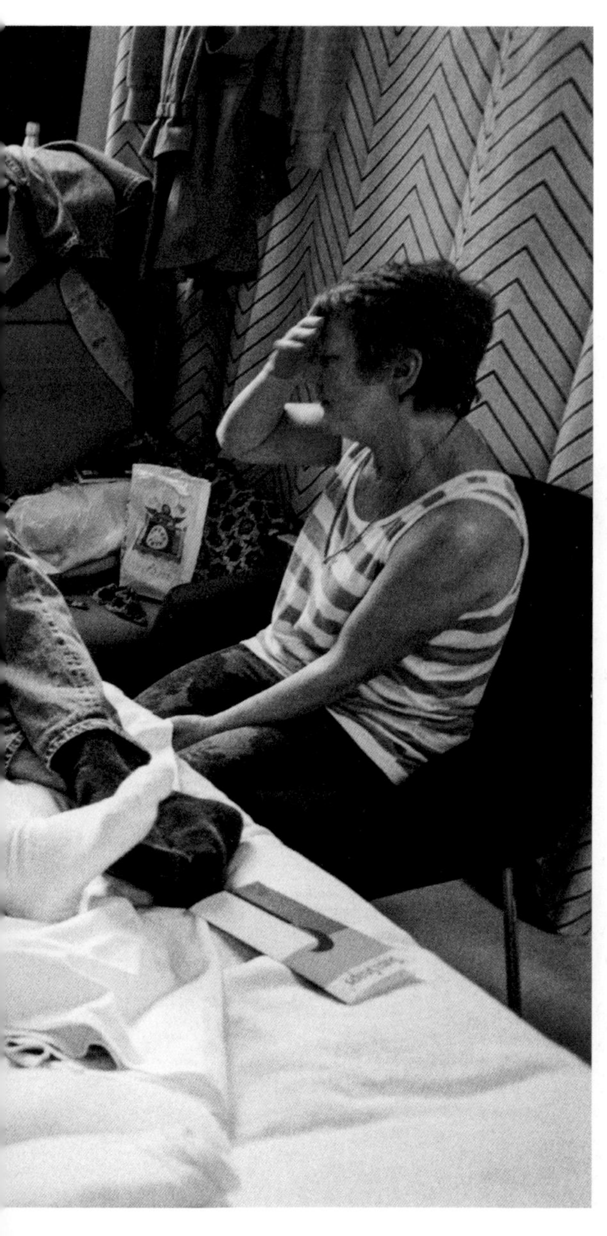

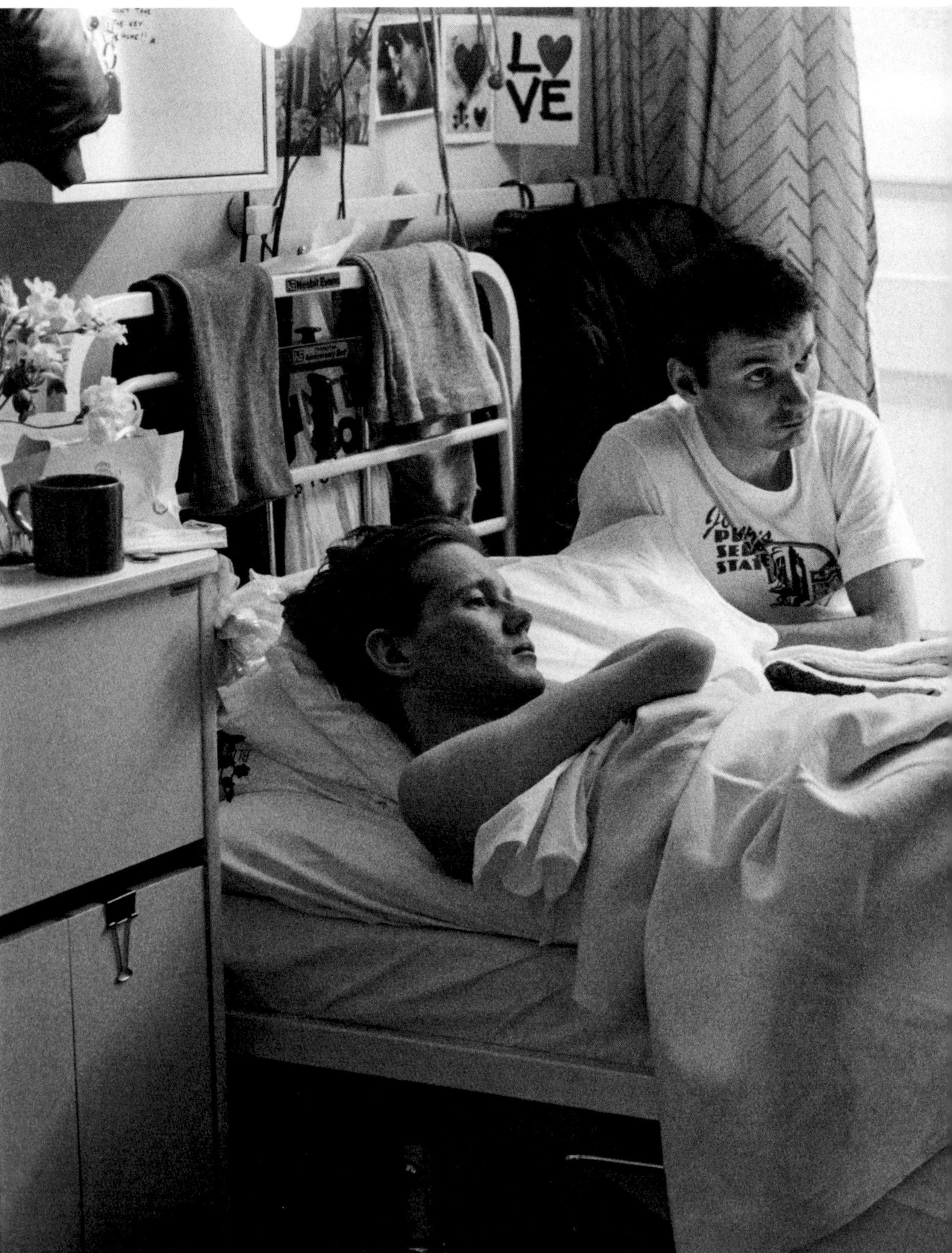
L♥
VE

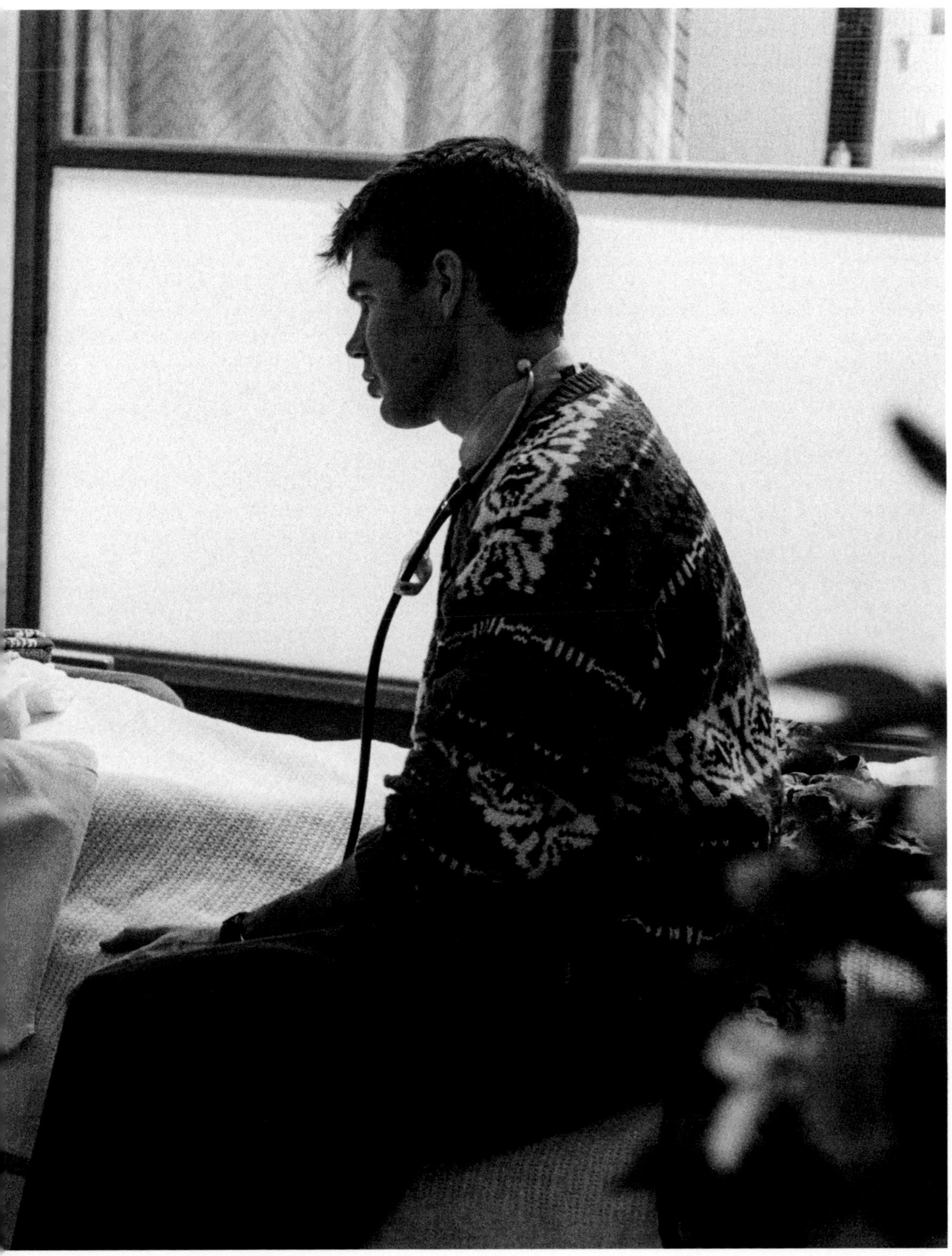

I was the Sister on Broderip Ward at the time. Our patients were mainly young gay men at the beginning of their lives. They were frightened, having seen many friends die already, and felt rejected and alone.

We tried to make the two in-patient wards (Broderip and Charles Bell) a place of warmth, safety and love. Life outside of the wards and the HIV clinic was hostile. Stigma was rife, fuelled by fear, ignorance and the media. In this climate, it was the HIV nurses' and doctors' role to protect the confidentiality of our in-patients on the wards, one slip on our part could result in patients being rejected by family or friends, being sacked or even an exposé in the press. We made sure the ward had nothing that could identify it was an HIV ward; the plaque marking the opening of the ward by Princess Diana was covered up by a painting and HIV information leaflets and posters were kept hidden in the nurses' rest room. This stigmatising extended to the staff, we would not always tell friends or family where we worked for fear of a hostile reaction. To make the ward a safe and welcoming space went beyond protecting confidentiality. I wanted to create a home-like environment.

We had subdued lighting, duvets on the beds; one patient had a large bowl of fish on his locker and scatter cushions in his room, much to the consternation of the Senior Nurse team in the Trust. I encouraged nurses to greet the patients with a hug as you would at home because many patients had been deprived of human touch because of 'fear of contamination'. We also enabled partners or family to stay overnight on a mattress on the floor in the patients' rooms if that was what the patient wished: All things that are part of showing true human compassion.

So, when Gideon approached me for permission to photograph the ward as part of the Positive Lives project, celebrating the 10th anniversary of the Terrence Higgins Trust, the answer had to be no. I felt we couldn't risk making the ward public when we had striven for years to maintain its anonymity. Although he assured me of the consent process for individual patients wishing to take part, I was concerned for all those past, current and future patients whose relatives, friends or colleagues would recognise the ward and staff in the photos and their cover would be blown. The price seemed too high. However, after several meetings we agreed for him to spend time on the ward in the background watching how the wards work and to reassure us that he would not be intrusive. It was clear from this that his approach was subtle, empathic and would probably help the fight against stigma rather than add to it. Thank goodness Gideon persuaded me because that early visual record has been captured for time to come. The collection complements the oral history of patients, staff and carers that we are now gathering to ensure we can learn from our experiences for now and in the future.

I feel so privileged to have been the ward sister of Broderip at that time, and remain moved and inspired by the resilience of the patients and their significant others, and the compassion and resolve of the staff.

**Jane Bruton,
Sister on Broderip ward, 1993**

Three weeks before Princess Diana was due to open the Broderip Ward in 1987, I got a panicked call from a Union leader at the hospital. No one had told the orderlies, porters, cleaning and kitchen staff about the new AIDS ward. Fear and stigma was rife and every household in the country had just received the AIDS: Don't Die of Ignorance leaflet. Some staff were threatening to boycott the ward, putting its opening in doubt. I went to a hastily arranged meeting in a smoke-filled basement room in the hospital. Many of the staff said that while they wanted to work on the ward, their families were fearful they would bring AIDS home with them. After three hours talking about the real routes of HIV transmission and how standard, hospital wide infection control would keep them and their families safe, the boycott was called off.

By 1993, the ward had cared for so many people with AIDS. Every year, the number of AIDS deaths continued to rise and, in remembrance, THT organised an annual Candlelight Memorial in

Trafalgar Square. I spoke that year, starting by saying "In the past four weeks, three friends have died one more has gone into hospital." I knew I was far from alone in experiencing this and that we needed a more permanent record of the extraordinary acts of love, caring, kindness and courage shown in response to this terrible epidemic. Positive Lives, published later that year, is now an essential part of that record. There were the real stories of use, gay lives, grief and loss, and it is fitting that Gideon Mendel's photos of the ward is the final chapter. With great sensitivity, he captured life on the ward and the ground-breaking way in which staff, patients, and their friends & families worked together to transform how great care can be delivered in the most challenging circumstances.

This approach, radical at the time, is now standard practice in much of the NHS. It is just one example of how our response to AIDS, born of fear, pain, love & loss, continues to reverberate throughout health & social care. It is salutary, though, that while most of the AIDS wards in London have now closed, there are more people living with HIV here than ever before. There is still so much more to be done.

Sir Nick Partridge,
Terrence Higgins Trust,
1985 - 2013

My Life Partner (Robert, 32, architect) was diagnosed with HTLV3 in 1982. When the test was introduced in 1984 I tested positive, and the doctor said: "Well, we're not surprised are we?" He gave me two years to live. I was going to die. That was it. There was nothing the doctors could do. No support networks, no counselling, no advice. You tried to live your life as best you could and you fought, how you fought! prejudice, ignorance, and for your rights. You started support groups and fund-raised and tried to raise awareness.

Robert passed away on New Year's Eve 86/87. Hundreds of people came to his funeral – doctors, nurses, friends, colleagues, and a tutor from his old university in South Africa. But not one of his family!

And then I was hospitalised... with pneumonia. I was on Charles Bell with a caring, supportive team around me. I once cried myself to sleep because I so wished my partner had had the same care. Then came the news that it wasn't PCP, just ordinary pneumonia and despite being extremely weak, after several days with the help of a nurse I was walking again. I also realised that I was not going to die.

I started visiting Broderip Ward - opened by Princess Diana but the brass plaque commemorating this momentous event was now hidden from view by flowers to avoid anyone actually knowing that this was the AIDS ward. Self stigma had started. I talked to people who might never leave the ward... skeletons in pain from sores and KS ... talked to people who had no visitors because they had been abandoned by friends and family...talked to people who despaired because they believed the clap trap about God's revenge and the gay plague... talked to people who had been victims of violence, abuse, prejudice, ignorance and discrimination. One boy had had his flat set on fire by neighbours so the council moved him... and the flat had a little garden for his cat... he came home one day and the cat had been hanged!

Terrible suffering... terrible despair... and yet the doctors and nurses carried on as professionally, positively and cheerfully as possible. In private they often shared their despair because they could do nothing for their patients... I remember one doctor crying on my shoulder because he was about to lose another patient. At the same time... there was hope... new medication was just around the corner. Wasn't it? 1996 was the turning point. Antiretroviral therapy was introduced. HIV became a manageable chronic disease rather than a death sentence. The more people who took therapy, the fewer people died. The newly diagnosed were suddenly being told they had a future.

Year after year I just kept on going. I turned out to be an exception to the rule. I had been given two years to live in 1984 and I managed to keep going without medication until 2003. I have now been living with the virus for 33 years and I am fit, healthy, in work and have a future.

**Chris Sandford,
former patient on Broderip
and Charles Bell wards**

Learning what to do when you don't know, what to do. Despite increasing knowledge, it was a time of crisis and of uncertainty – many people were very sick and were dying. Learning how to work with not knowing was an important skill as even the most experienced of clinicians found themselves seeing something for the first time. It was a continuous exercise in using first principles to make an accurate diagnosis. Paying careful attention to the patient's story, carrying out meticulous physical examinations, taking blood and tissue samples for laboratory analysis wherever they might give a clue to the underlying problem that could then guide treatment.

Medicine for HIV itself was just beginning. AZT was the first and at that time only drug available. It had been shown to give some additional time to people with AIDS. We were learning how it should best be used, and how to help people deal with its side effects, which were often extremely debilitating. Research was an integral part of the work, with the hospital leading a major research trial (the Concorde Study) to see if people could gain any benefit from taking AZT in the earlier stages of infection. The results suggested not.

It seems, looking back, that boundaries between us all were more blurred than in other

areas of medicine. We found ways to share our
feelings about what was going on around us. We
developed ways of working that allowed us to share
intelligence with others who had more experience,
to exchange data and to link treatment activists
and patients with other sources of information and
expertise. I frequently witnessed the considerable
fear, stigma, isolation and loneliness that people
with HIV experienced. That many were unable
to tell others about their HIV infection added
another dimension. Right the way through, the
interelationships between the biomedical, the
social and the political responses were always
startlingly clear and made a strong impression.

It was a very influential period both personally
and professionally, and a privilege to work in this
area of medicine and to have experienced being a
small part of the team at the Middlesex Hospital.

Dr Jane Anderson,
senior registrar at Middlesex Hospital
1988 - 1990

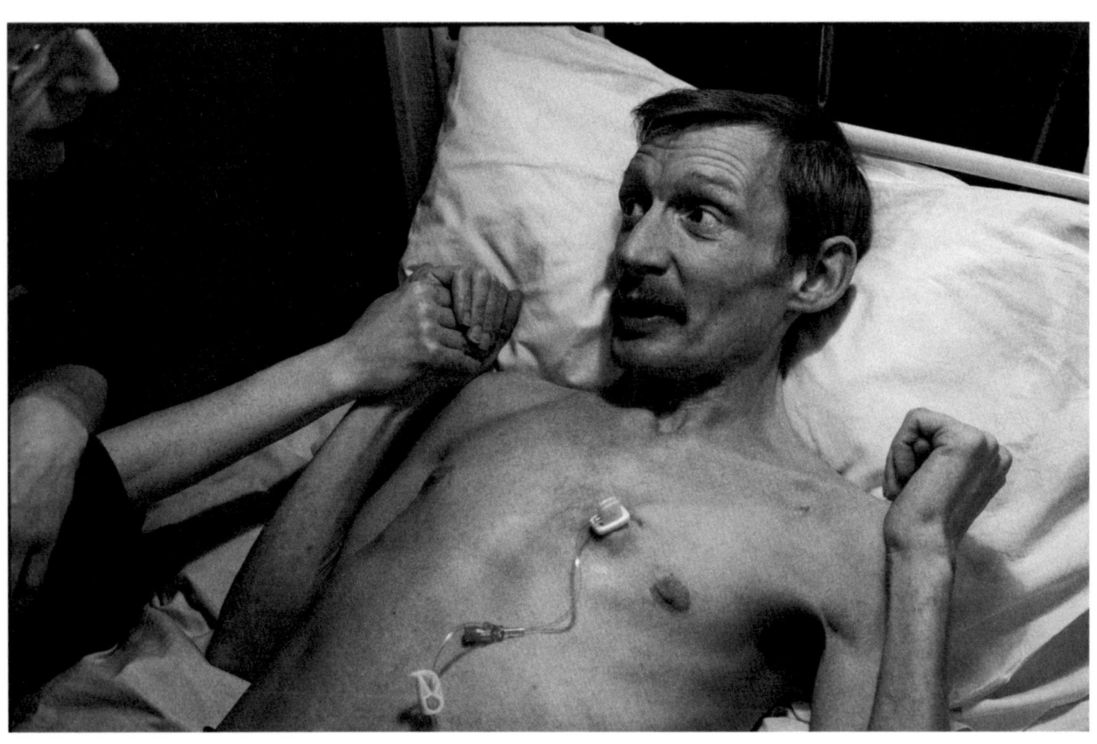

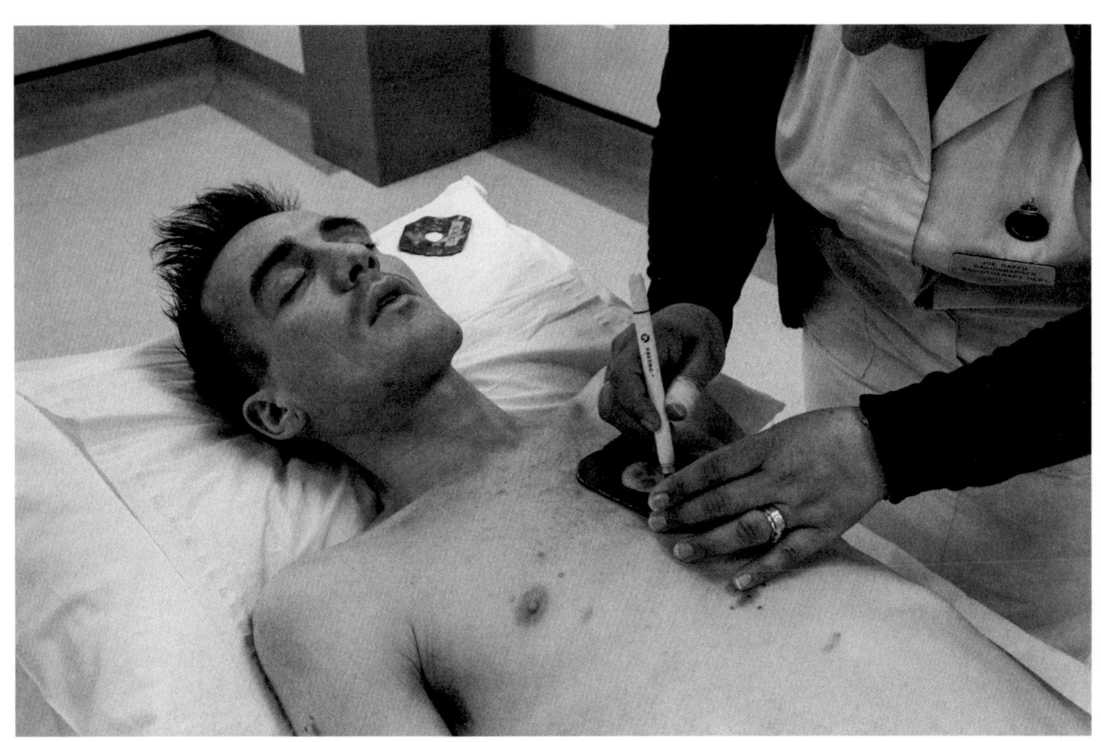

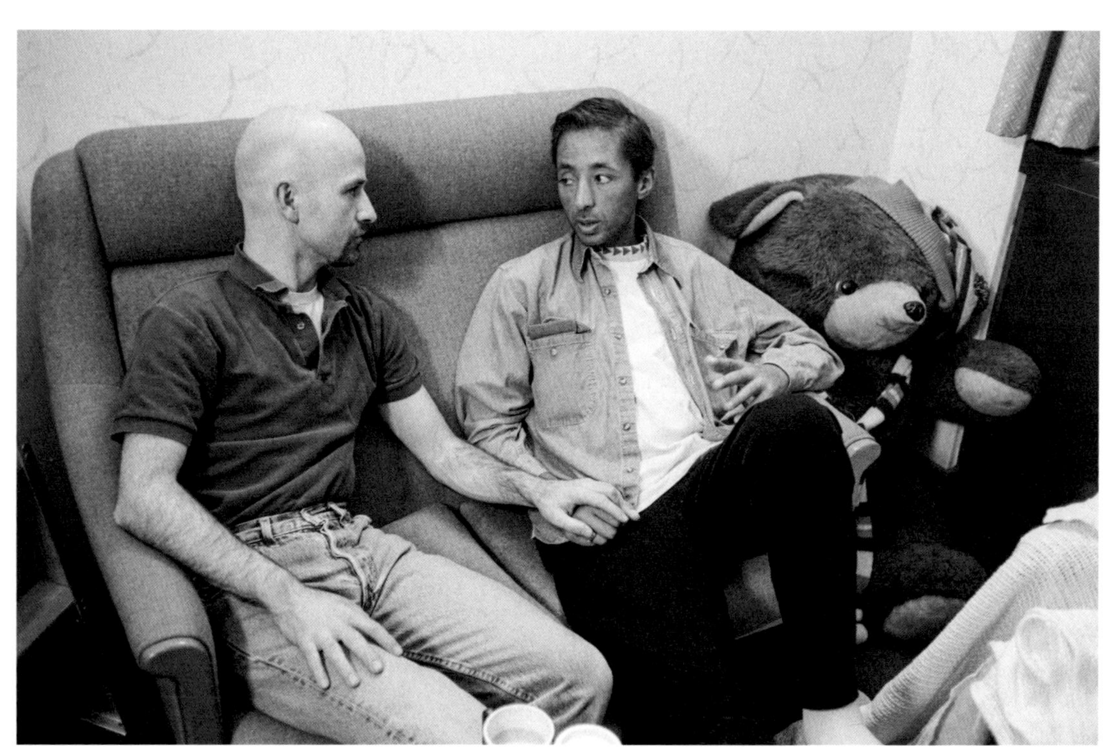

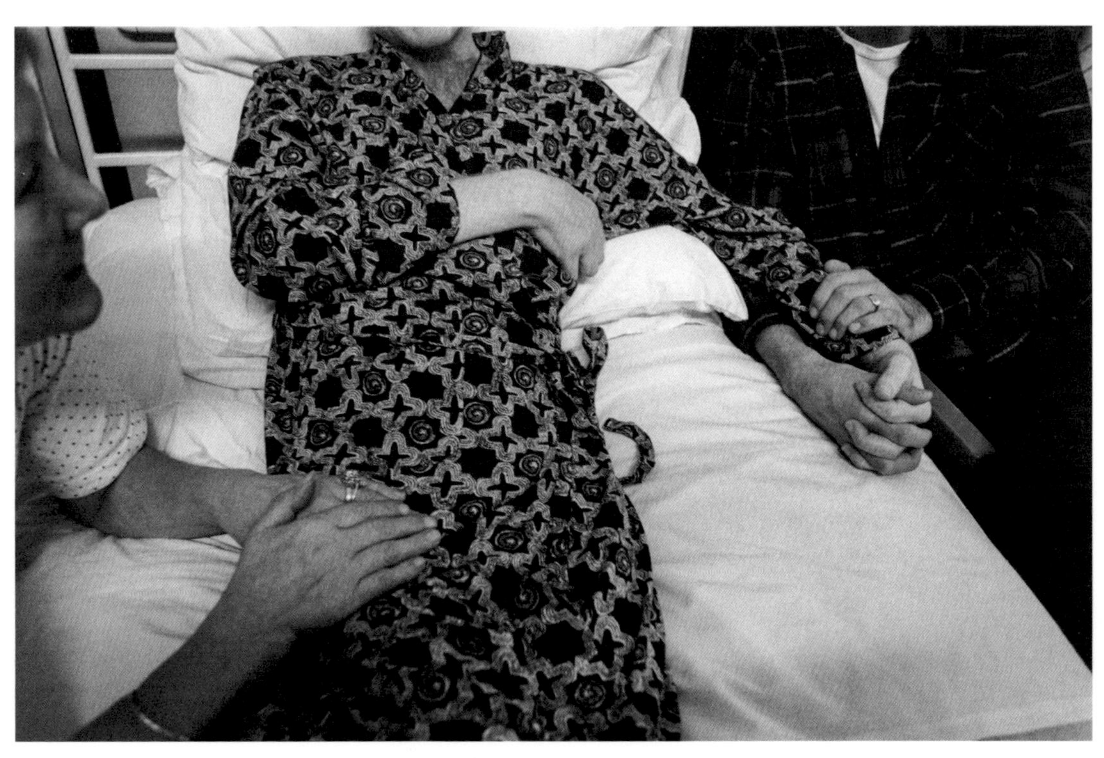

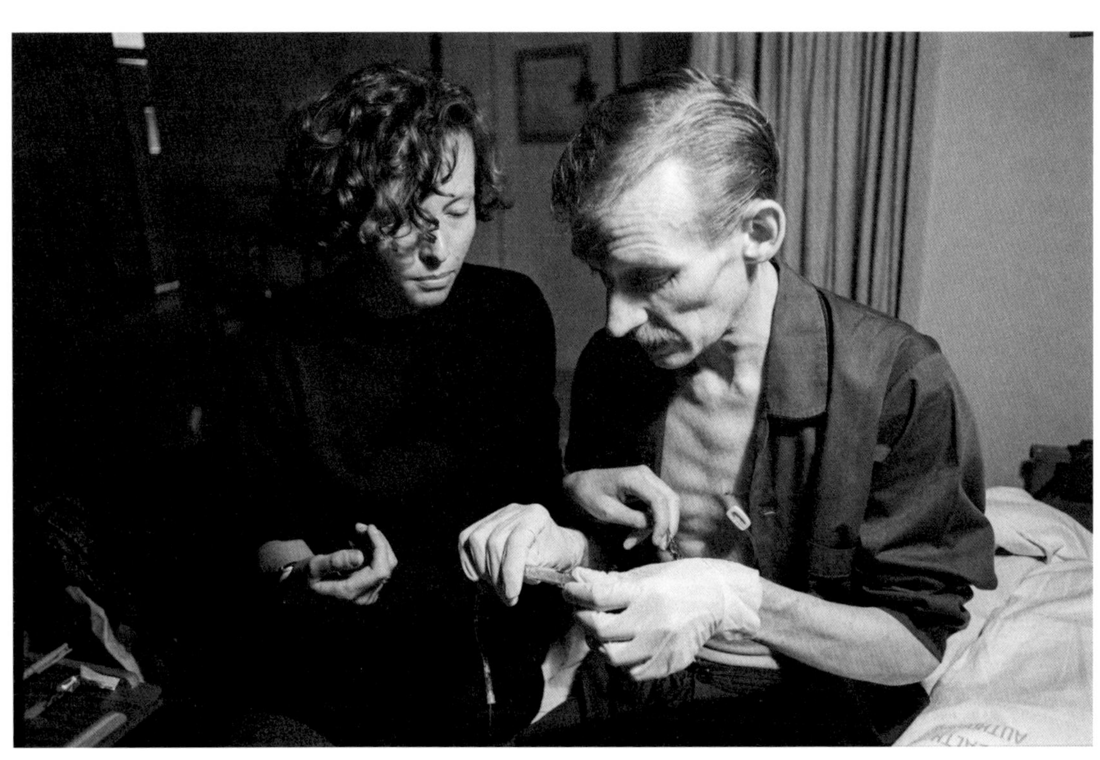

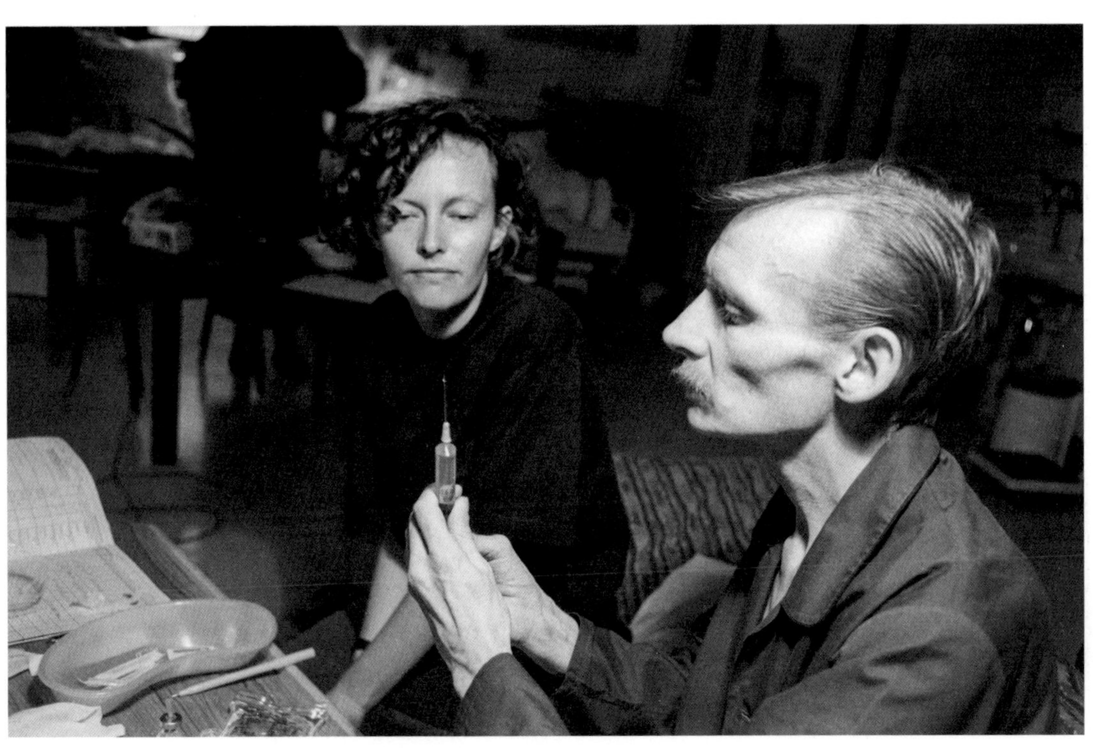

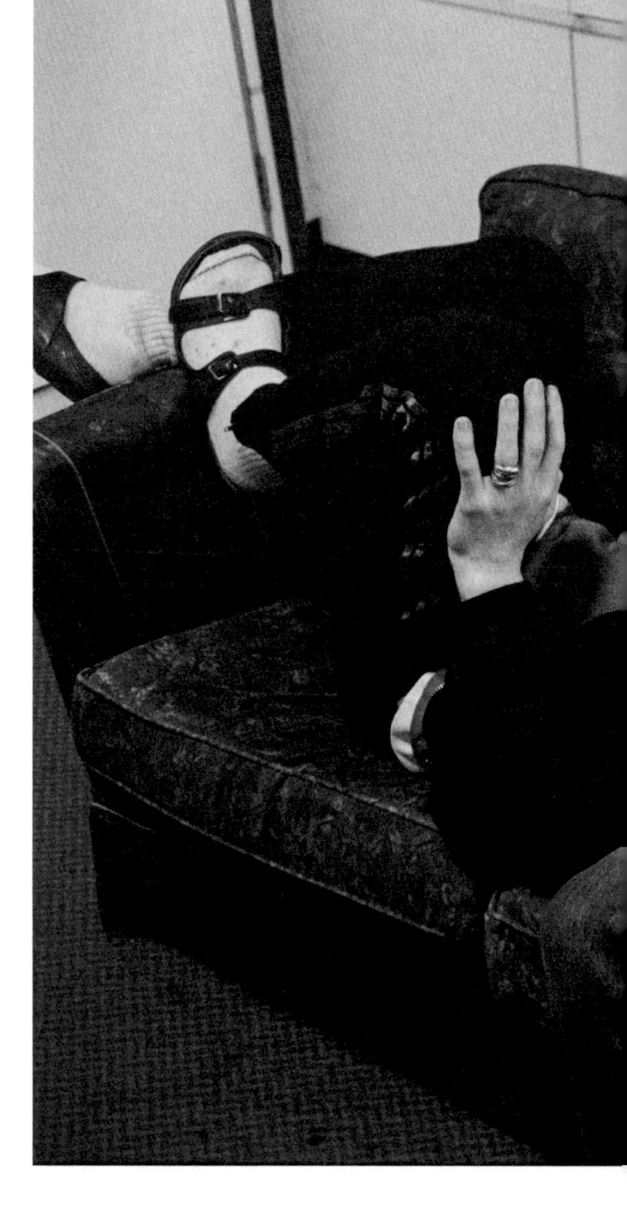

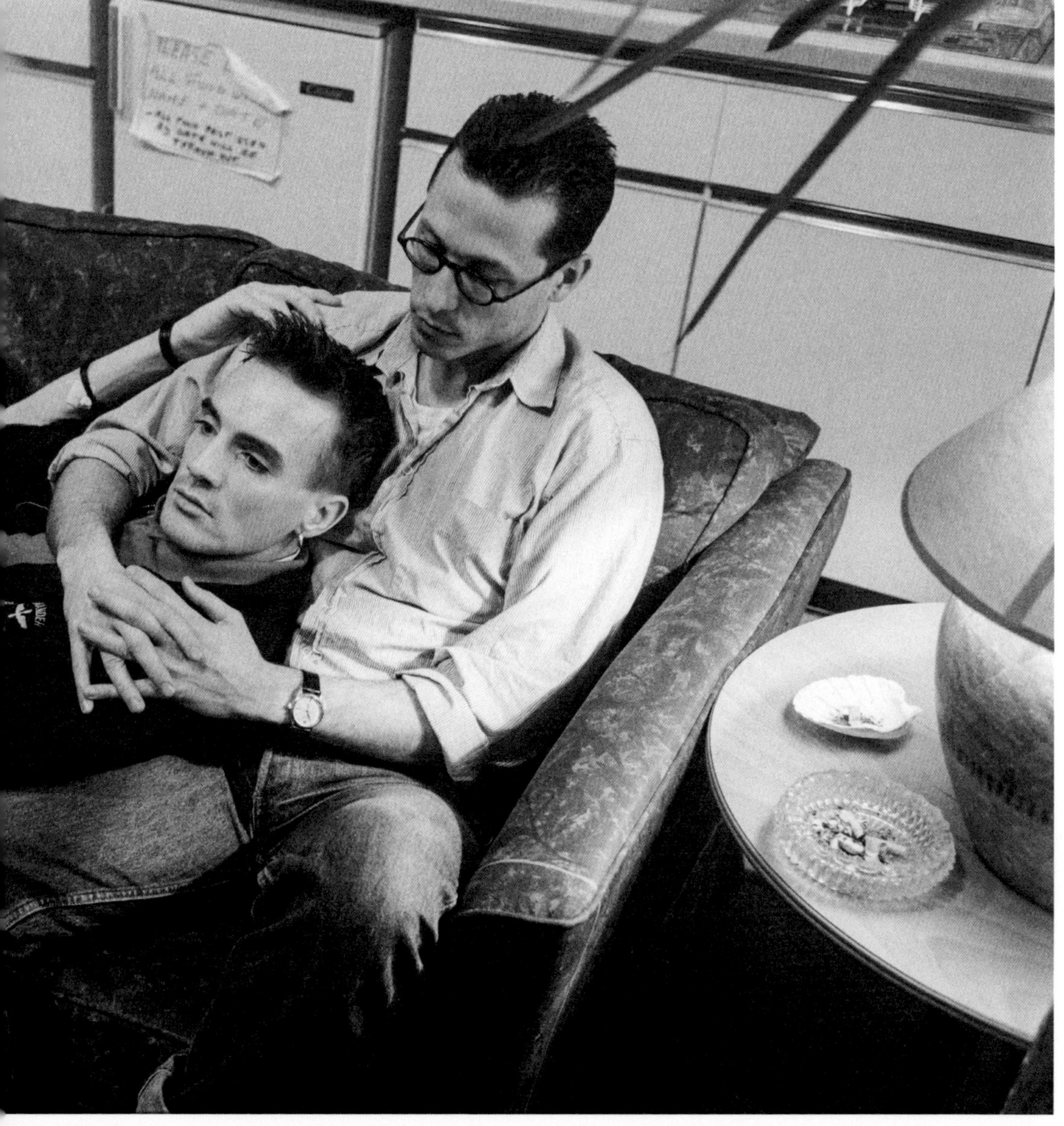

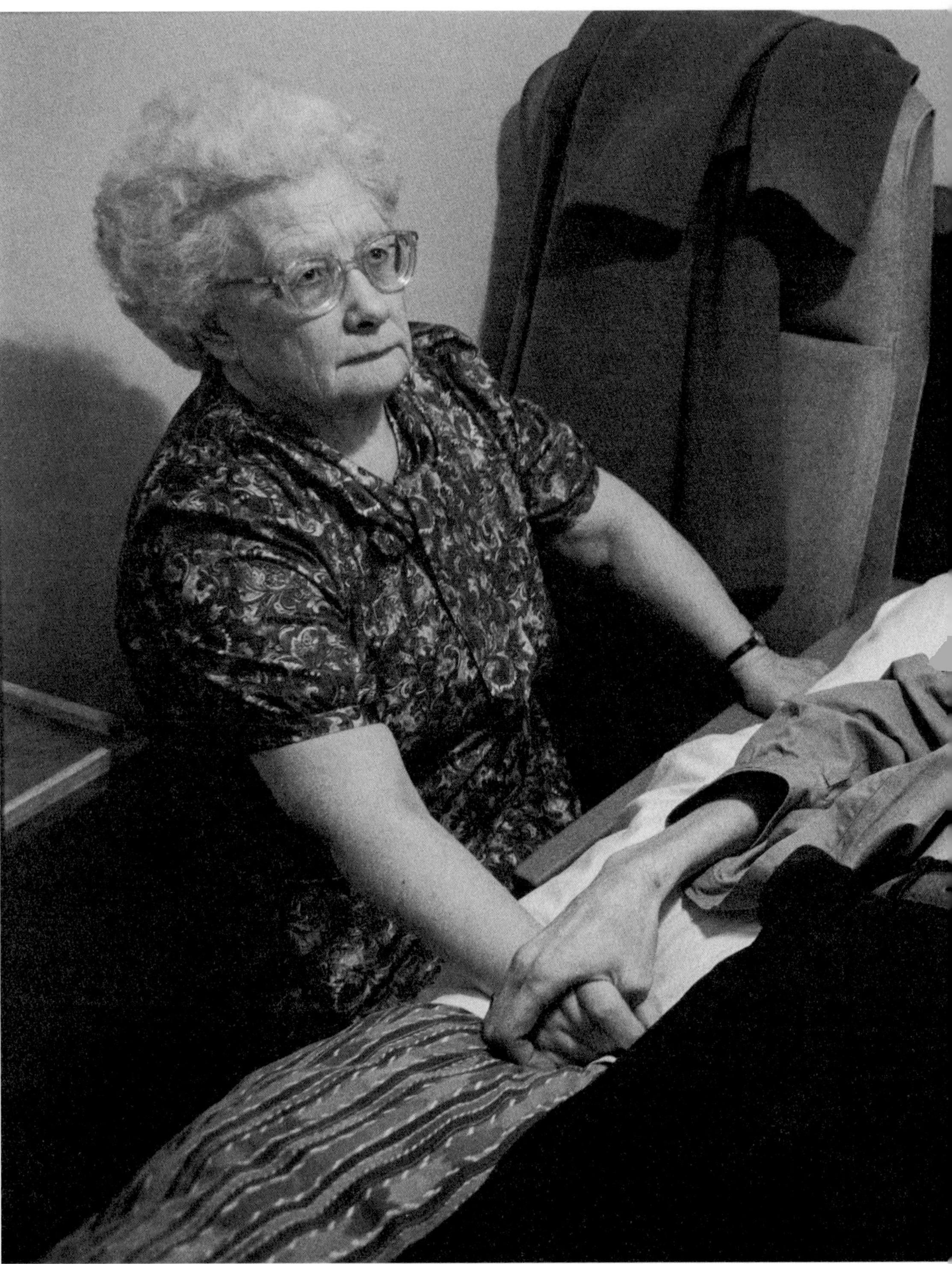

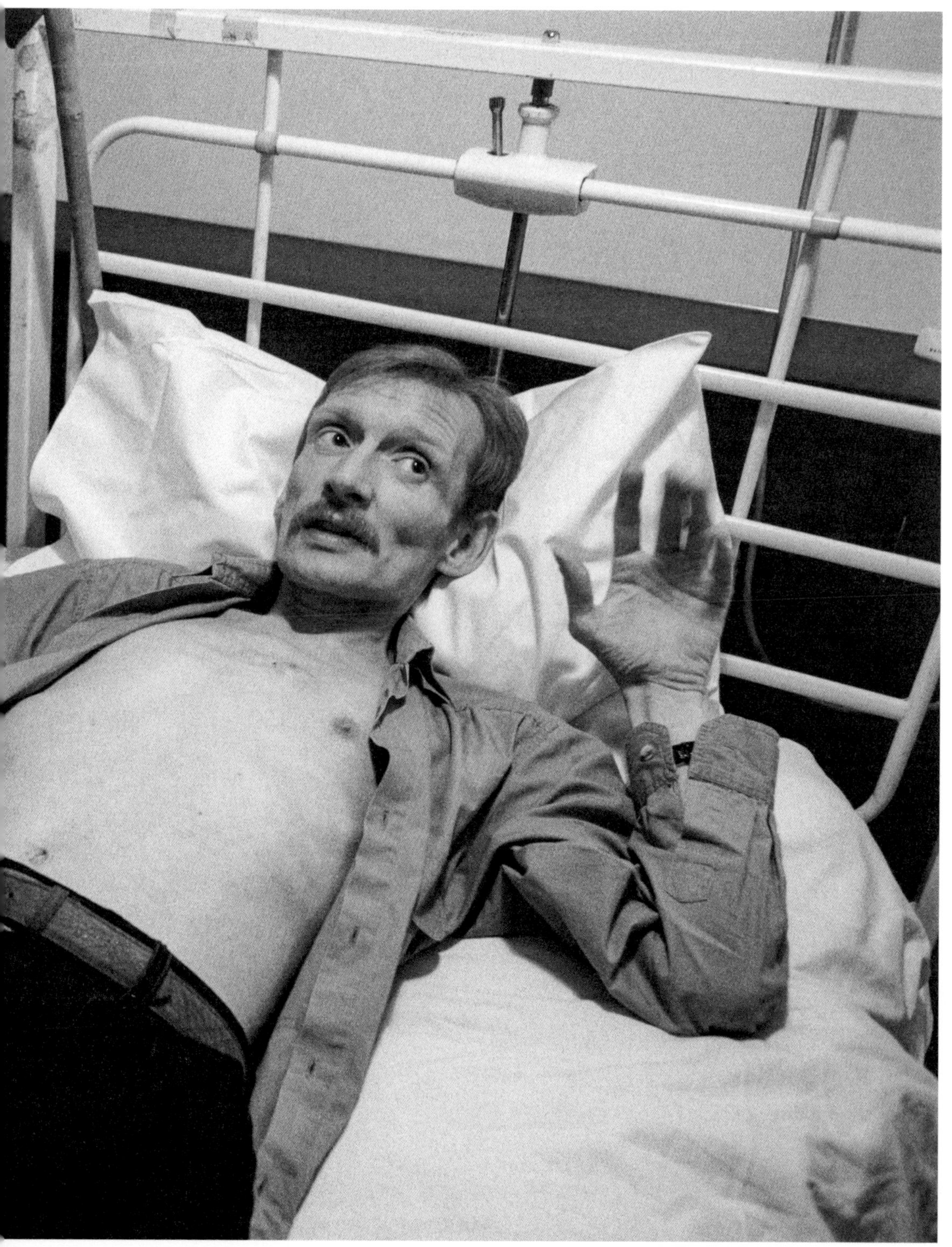

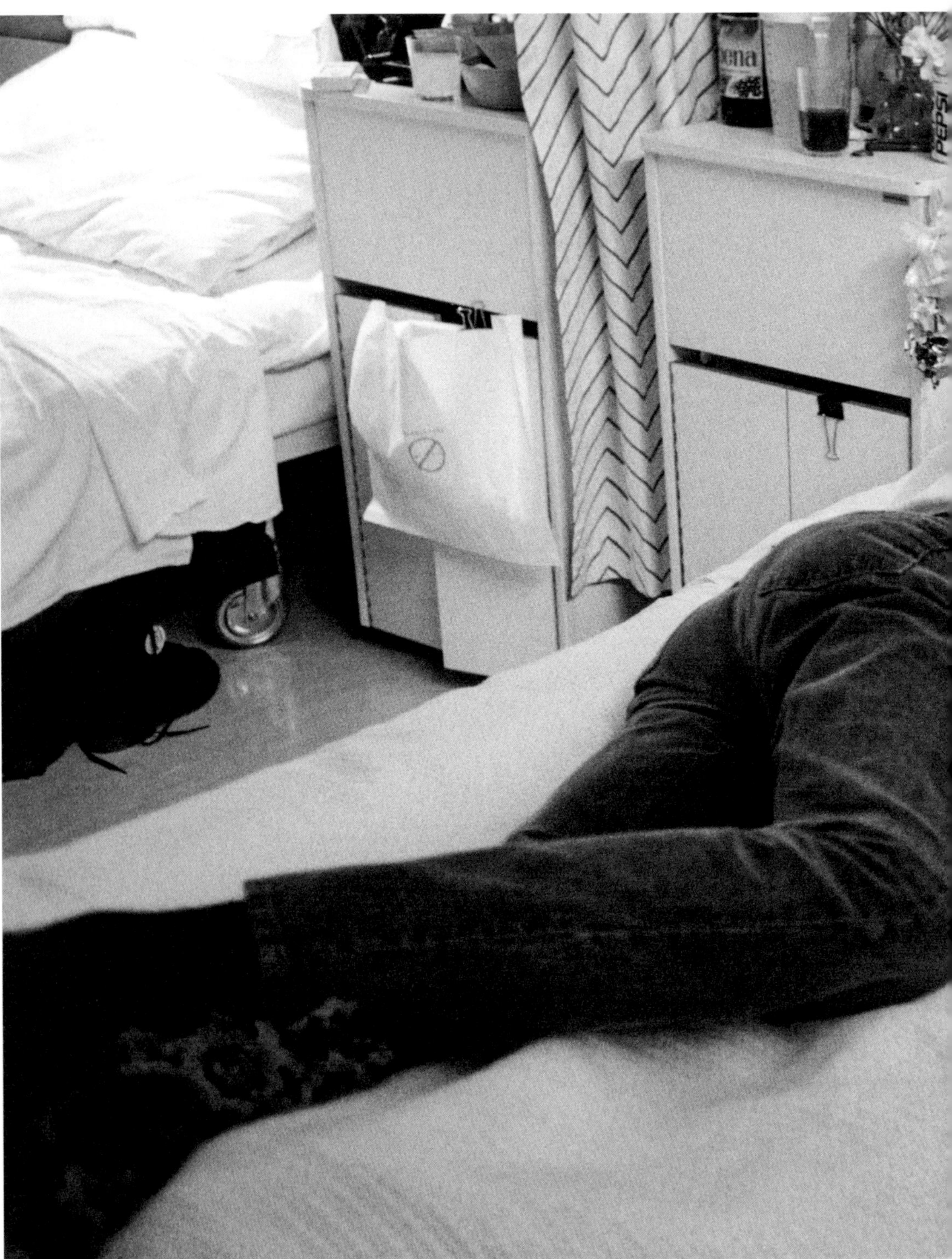

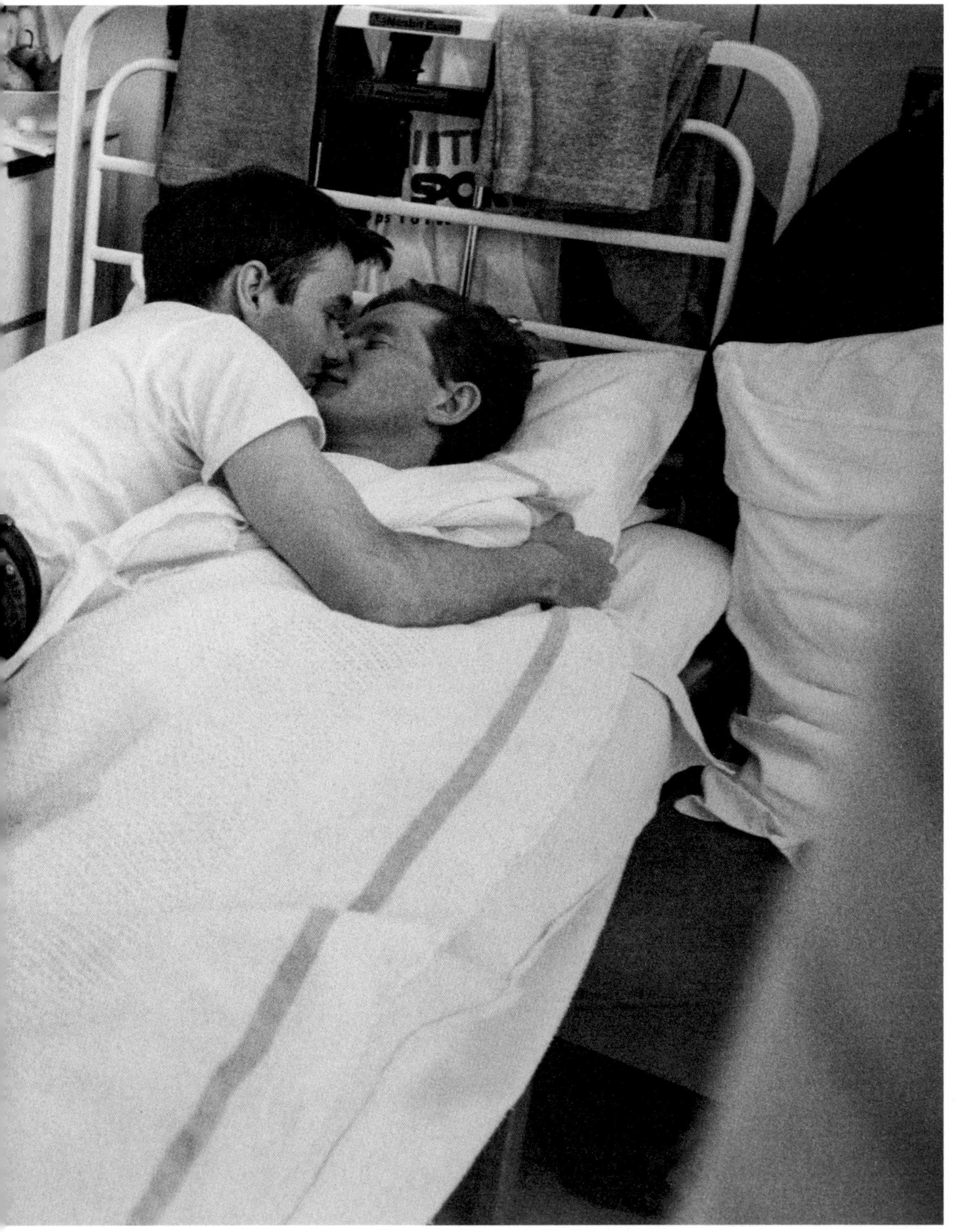

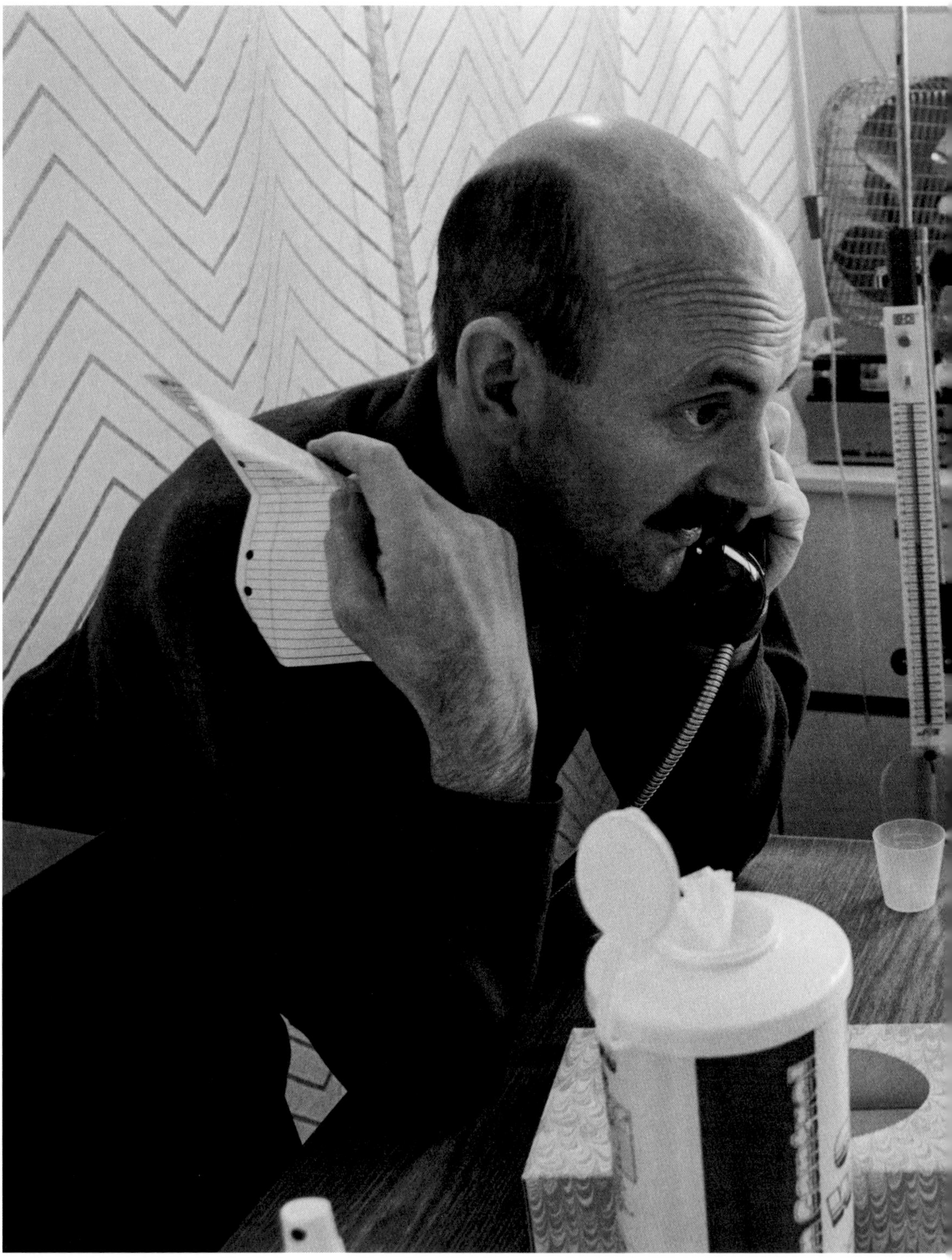

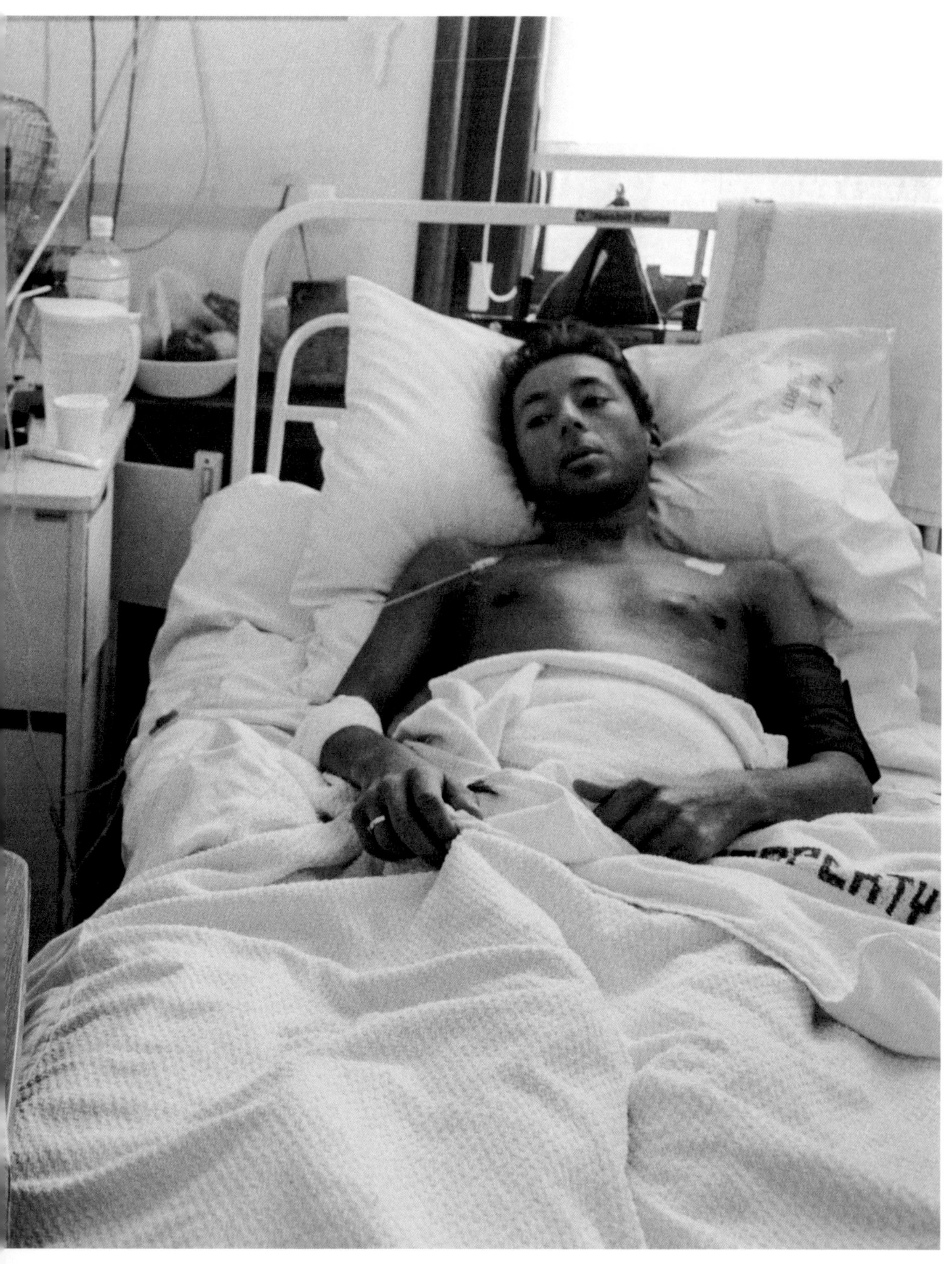

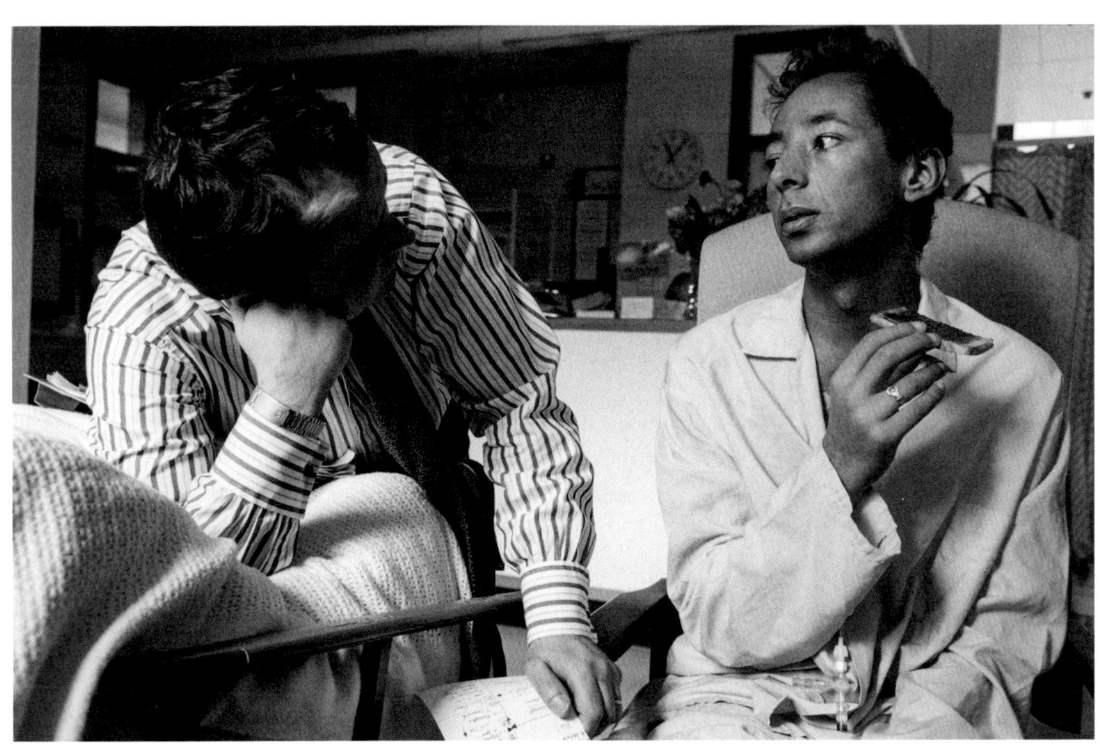

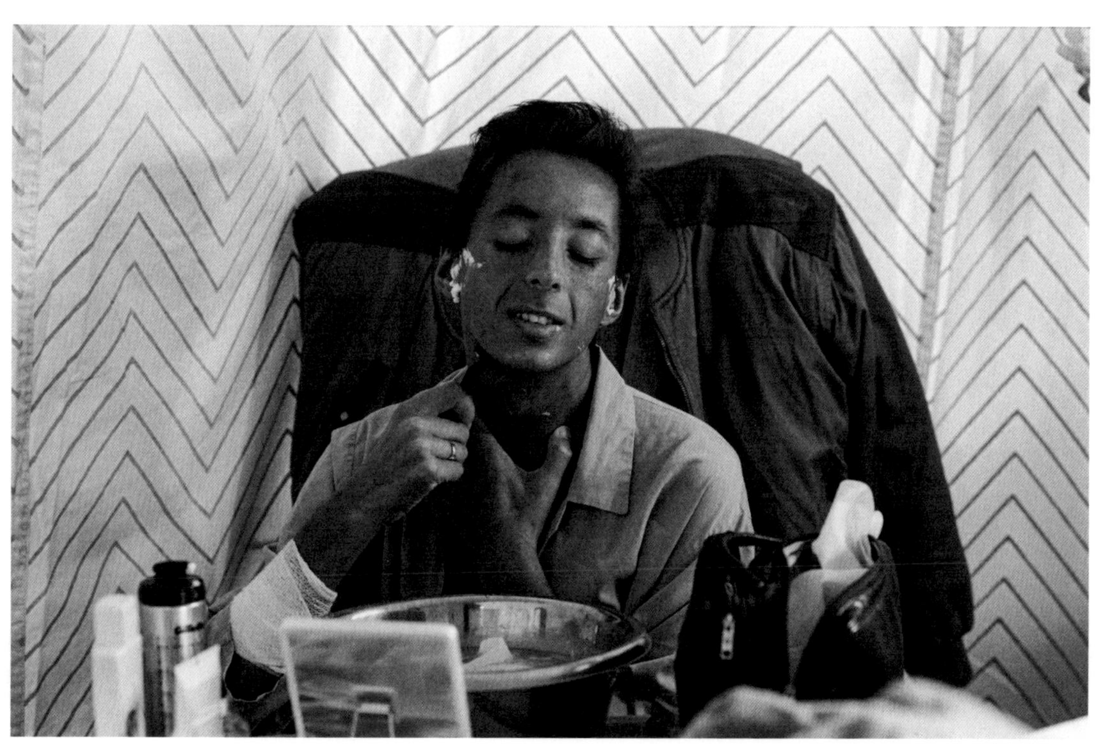

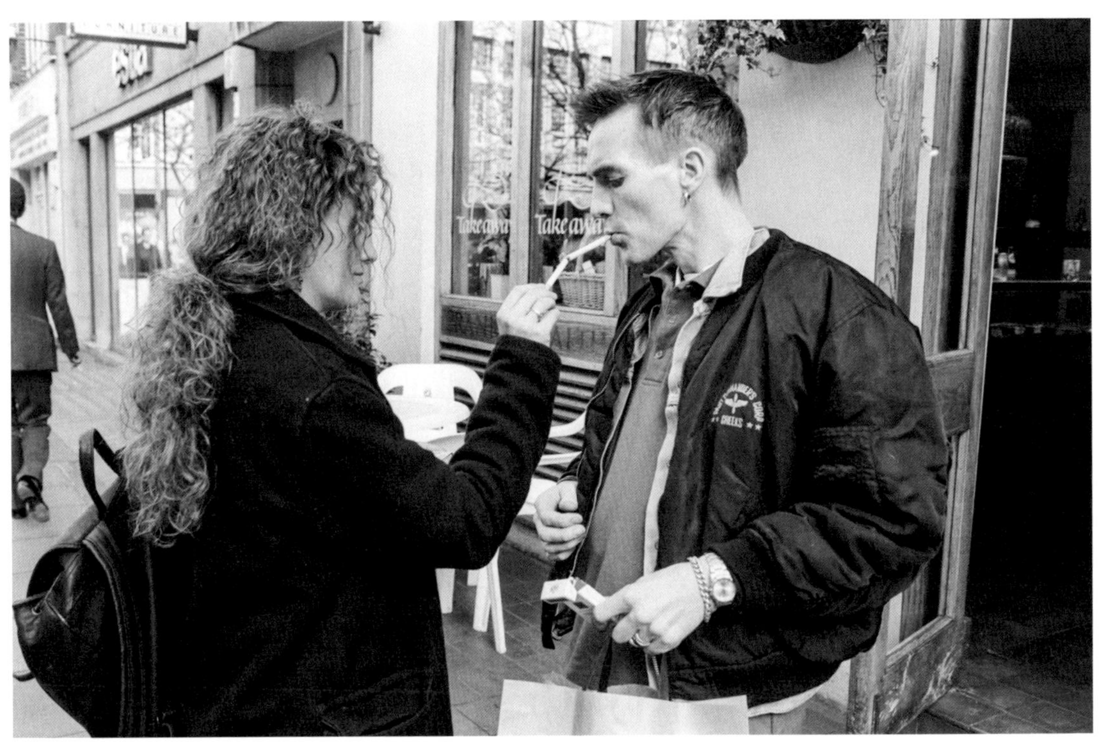

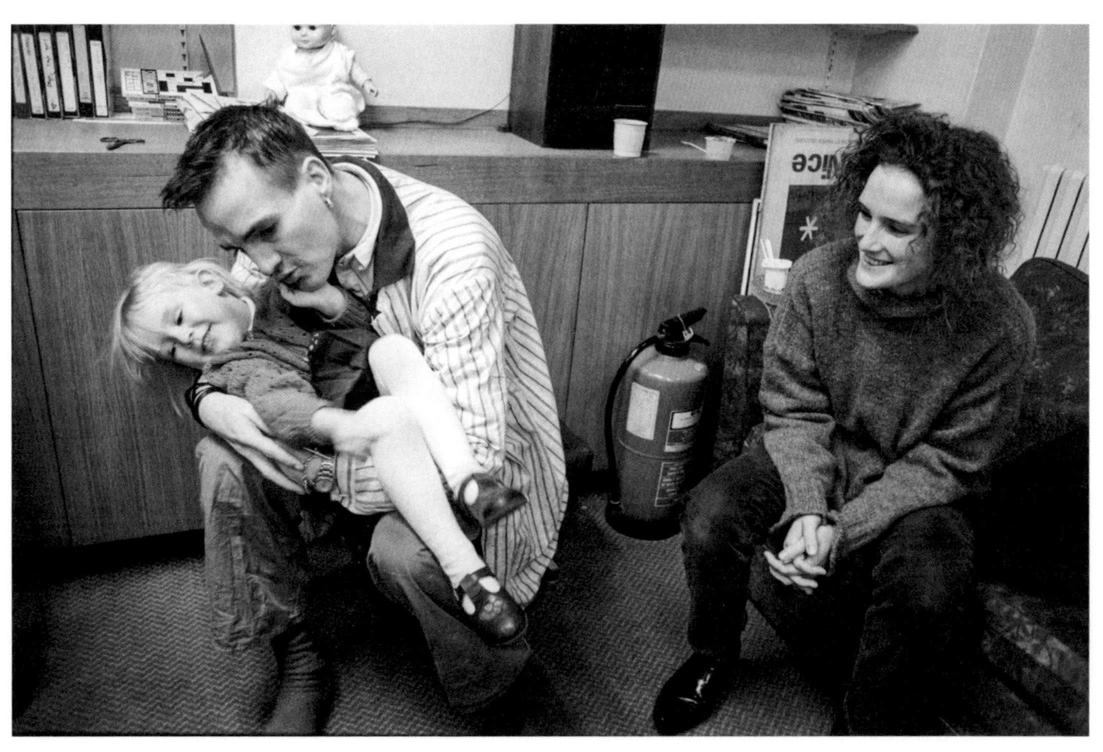

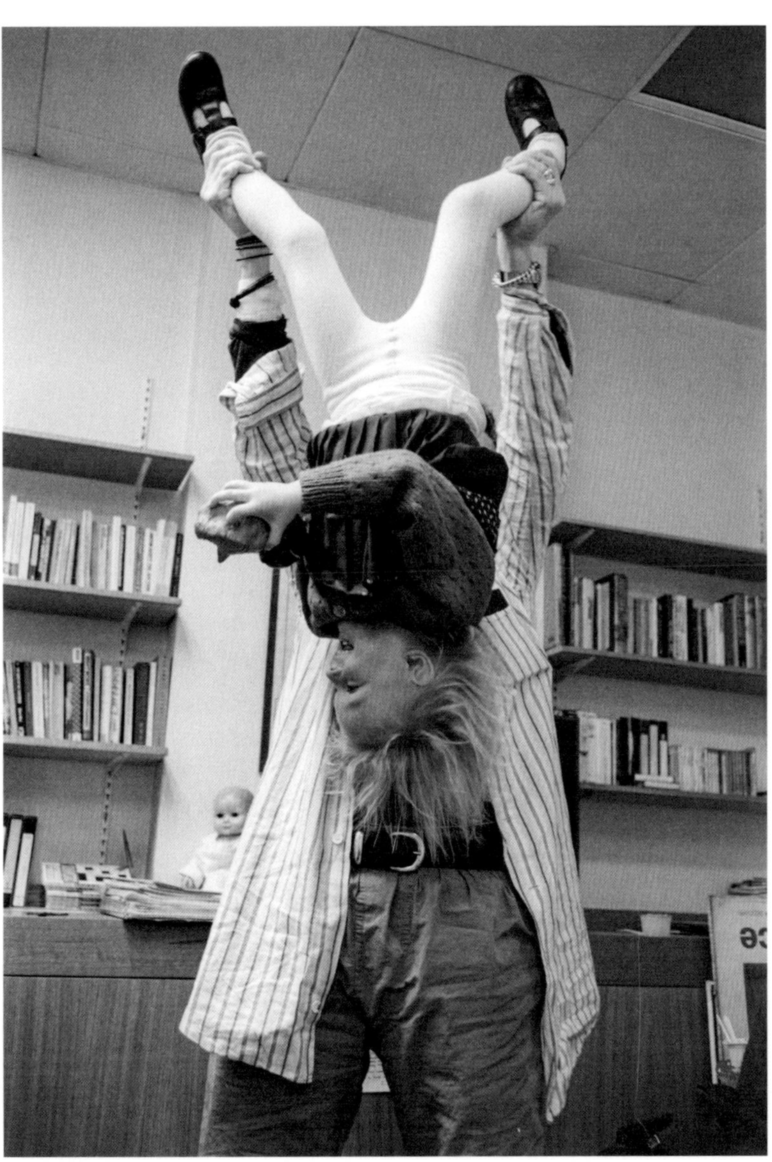

24 years to the day of Steven's death on Oct 1st 1993, I'm writing these few words.

During my visits to Steven's private room on Broderip ward we would often lay on the bed in each other's arms. We often fell asleep that way at any time of day. Mercurial angels resting their wings. In those days every time one woke up, reality, like the old fashioned railway departure boards, would rapidly shutter down it's unrelentingly harsh truths in one's mind and before one's eyes. Yes this most gruelling and yet most treasured of times was indeed happening.

It seemed strange at first to sleep with a friend on a hospital ward where I also had a professional presence as shiatsu support worker to the nursing team. But boundaries between staff and patients were, if at times existent at all, so often gossamer thin.

Some time into Steven's care on the ward a new nurse called Sarah appeared and was assigned to tend to Steven. From the outset, for no good reason I'm sure, he told her to fuck off. Somehow in his Belfast accent 'fuck off' always sounded as if it was being simultaneously struck in gold, a blessing as much as a curse. To his surprise and utter delight Sarah immediately turned to him and said, "No, do you know what? You fuck off!" From that moment, Steven and Sarah became the very closest of friends and allies in the combat of the disease and in the journey along the road to his death. Steven and Sarah's laughter together is one of the things I particularly remember. Yet strangely the thought of that laughter, so vital at the time to face the hard rain of those days, can bring tears to my eyes even now.

The most enduring memory I have from my time both working at and visiting friends on the ward followed a call from Steven to come to the hospital as he was undergoing a blood transfusion. Expecting the worst I raced to the ward. As I reached the top of the stairs, there he stood, barefoot in his pyjamas, attached to the mobile drip, in one hand he was waving a half bottle of brandy, in the other a fat joint, and through his inimitable laughter said, "We're blessing the blood darling! We're blessing the blood!" We drank a toast to the new blood together. It was not unusual to turn up at the ward for a visit only to be told Steven was shopping in Heal's across the road, or had gone out clubbing the night before and had not yet returned. His private room on Broderip served as a most convenient West End pied a terre.

Only this week in the U.S. the Center for Disease Control has announced its compliance with the campaign U=U, where an undetectable viral load means HIV is untransmittable. We live in such very different times.

Those we lost were our frontline soldiers. "They shall not grow old, as we that are left grow old." What purpose is there now in life that could ever match the shared purpose of those times, save to love and love and love again.

Chris Mazeika,
shiatsu therapist on the Broderip ward

I joined the staff of Broderip ward as a Lecturer in Medicine (senior trainee) in March 1987. It was the first purpose built HIV/AIDS ward in UK. It had opened its doors to patients in January that year, and was officially opened by Diana, Princess of Wales on 09 April. The same evening a "This Week" documentary entitled "The toughest job in medicine" presented by (Baroness) Margaret Jay was shown on ITV. Suddenly the ward was in the public's eye!

In 1987 no effective antiretroviral medication was available, and a diagnosis of HIV was effectively a death sentence. Broderip was a unique hospital environment. The ward team were decades ahead of the rest of the NHS at the time - in that we had a truly multi-disciplinary team of nurses, doctors, psychologists, social workers, physiotherapists, and housekeepers, all providing personalised care for the patients. We also championed our patients to take an active part in deciding their treatment plans. Indeed many patients were extremely knowledgeable about their illness, and its complications, and some knew more than we did! Many patients spent long periods on the ward, as their treatment was lengthy, others needed to be admitted many times, as their weakened immune system made them vulnerable to a plethora of infections. Over time the ward became almost a second home to many patients, as well to their partners and families. As a team we were privileged to be able to care for these young men, as well being able get to know them, and their families, as fellow human beings.

Over the last 30 years my professional career has focussed on providing care for people living with HIV and its complications. With hindsight, I think the title of Margaret Jay's documentary should have been "The most rewarding job in medicine"!

Professor Rob Miller,
Senior Registrar 1987
and Honorary Consultant 1991,
Broderip and Charles Bell wards

My first job as a qualified nurse was on Broderip. The sister who is now a good friend chuckles about the risk she took when she employed me as everyone else who worked there was very experienced indeed. I had no experience as a qualified staff nurse but I knew I wanted to work in a holistic setting.

It's hard to believe now but in the 80s 'holistic' wasn't commonly a consideration on medical wards in big hospitals. On Broderip, it was a matter of course. The unit operated a bit like an extended family - we were united by a desire to counteract the negative effects of HIV. They were frightening times for everybody really - but there was genuine bravery demonstrated by so many of the patients day after day. We had to be brave as staff too the attachment and loss cycle was profound.

I remember a day when Lady Di was due to visit - she was well loved and very popular on that ward. I opted to do the nightshift (I was too anti-royal to curtsy!) and colleagues told me later that day how much time she spent with the patients.

If I walk past the Middlesex hospital now, those days are unrecognisable. I feel sad that how we were nursing in the 80s and 90 is so hard to imagine now.

Dr Denise Barulis,
former nurse on Broderip ward

My brother Kennedy, or simply just 'K' as the family affectionately nicknamed him, died from AIDs related PCP (a form of pneumonia) complications in early 1995. He was only 32 years old. During the last three years of his life, 'K' spent a lot of time in and out of the Broderip Ward. He had every opportunistic infection going. He had TB, meningitis, Kaposi's sarcoma, epileptic fits, you name it. The Broderip became like a second home to him. And in some ways to me too. Although mum went to a lot of appointments with 'K', I took on the responsibility of visiting him whenever he was in the hospital. One of my lasting memories of visiting him there was the fact that what he wanted more than anything was a big hug as soon as I walked in and again when I left. I can't even begin to imagine what it must have been like for him to constantly be in and out of hospital and to witness fellow patients deteriorating and dying all around him. It must have been soul destroying. Thinking about it now, it is clear that he so needed to feel loved. And that hugs were clearly an important way for him to feel that he wasn't being rejected.

And so I was in and out of the Broderip whenever he was admitted. I didn't even realise how often I was in there until one of their former in-patients, whom I later met years later at a support group after I too was diagnosed with HIV, said to me, 'I used to see you at the Broderip all the time and actually thought that you worked there!' What struck me most about the Broderip ward was how welcoming, accommodating, relaxed and flexible the staff were. Other visitors and I could spend hours in there. Way past visiting times sometimes, but the staff just turned a blind eye.

From what I could see, the staff were more concerned about ensuring their patients were comfortable. And they understood that having family and friends around were invaluable to the patients. So they let us be.

To this day, I still remember the way the staff at the Broderip treated my brother. When all around us people were judging and stigmatising against people living with HIV, the staff at the Broderip continued to treat all their patients with care and compassion.

Angelina Namiba,
sister of former Broderip ward patient

Looking at the pictures now I am struck by how much hugging and touching there was. Maybe it was because there was little treatment and the stigma was terrible. Touch became so much part of our caring. I remember when doing nights having intense late night conversations with the patients. These young men felt guilty and blamed themselves. It was awful.

It was not all sad. During the day there was a particular intense energy in the ward. Everybody knew our patients were dying and every moment was charged with bravado and bravery. Something very honest was going on. It was so different to every other nursing experience. Young men were planning their own funerals, deciding how it should be done. It was inspiring to see those patients take control of their own life and death.

Steven taught me so much. He died soon after we took these photographs. I remember his franticness and determination to live life when he knew he was dying. He fitted pads under his T-shirts so he could carry on going out. He continued living and travelling to the end.

I was a young nurse and I was dealing with overwhelming issues that I did not really understand. Thinking about it now, I can see that when you are in this situation you can either step back and not do anything or step too far forward. Coming so close to my patients was my natural response. It was all a bit much, but it was absolutely the right thing to do at that time. Often we don't do enough. Getting the right balance is an art that you learn.

That experience taught me something very important about caring. I was so lucky to have worked there for that brief time. It shaped the rest of my life.

Sarah Macauley,
staff nurse on Broderip ward,
1992 - 1994

Stevie Whitson was one of the greatest lighting designers I ever worked with. He'd lit Andy Warhol's play "Pork" at La Mama in New York and moved to Britain after having kicked drugs in a methadone clinic in Ireland. He shaped my taste and made me look at art and theatre differently. He'd become

very ill in Russia and by the time I regularly visited
him at the Broderip ward in the Middlesex Hospital,
he was dying. His bed was right in the centre of the
ward. I remember walking through and running
the gauntlet with men who smiled and were friendly,
but who looked so very ill. They almost always had
visitors though and the atmosphere was ribald and
lively, friendly, inclusive and very open. It wasn't
what you'd expect in a ward which for many was
terminal. Stevie did not look that ill and every time
I went in, I secretly hoped he'd rally and leave.
He told me that a couple of the patients had started
relationships with each other whilst on the ward
too. That openness and inclusivity was what struck
me every time I visited. The nurses were extraordin-
arily warm and empathic. Certainly the nurse who
was Stevie's primary carer seemed to understand
his needs in an intuitive, umbilical way. He and
photographer Mike Goldwater had discussed
working together on images for Lyndall Stein's
ground-breaking book "Positive Lives", but Stevie
died before the ideas he'd formulated could come
to fruition. I worried that his amazing legacy would
be forgotten, but Hollywood director, Mike Figgis,
who'd worked with Stevie in his early UK theatre
days, visited the ward often too. He later made a
film about Stevie's death and cast him as a kinetic
theatre visionary portrayed by Robert Downey Jr.
I think Stevie would have liked that. I found out, only
a couple of weeks ago, that Toynbee Studio have
named their largest dance studio after him too. So I
guess he isn't forgotten. When I think of him now, I
think of visiting him on that ward. It wasn't a place
of peace or quiet. It was not like any other ward I
have been to since where people are very ill. There
was an extraordinary energy, noise, strength and
life to the ward. It was almost as if the patients
demanded that vigour. The nurses and doctors
responded with a space which was not conservative
or controlling, unlike so many other hospital wards.

**Robert Chevara,
friend of Stevie Whitson, former patient**

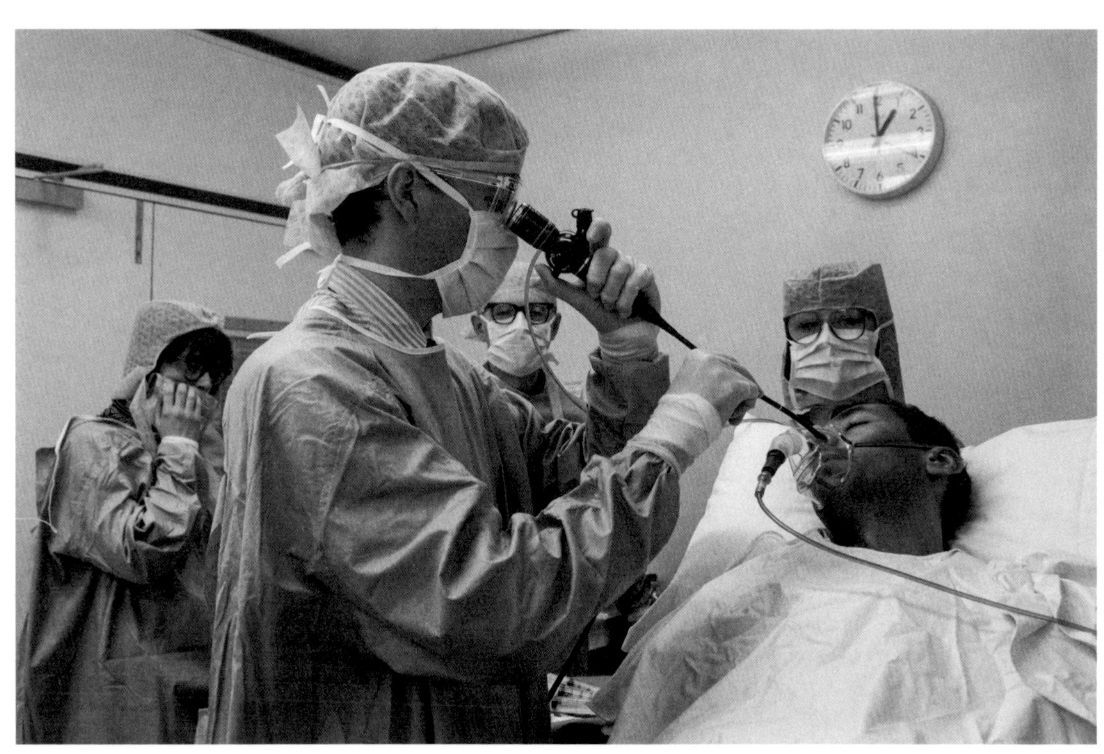

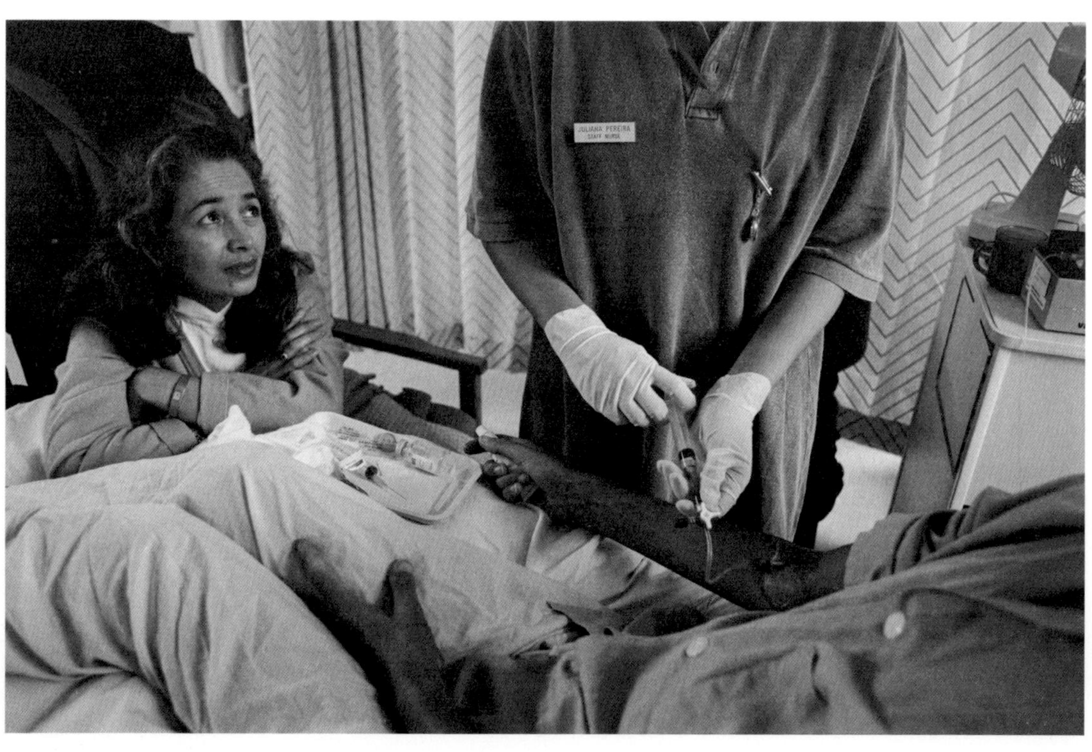

JULIANA PEREIRA
STAFF NURSE

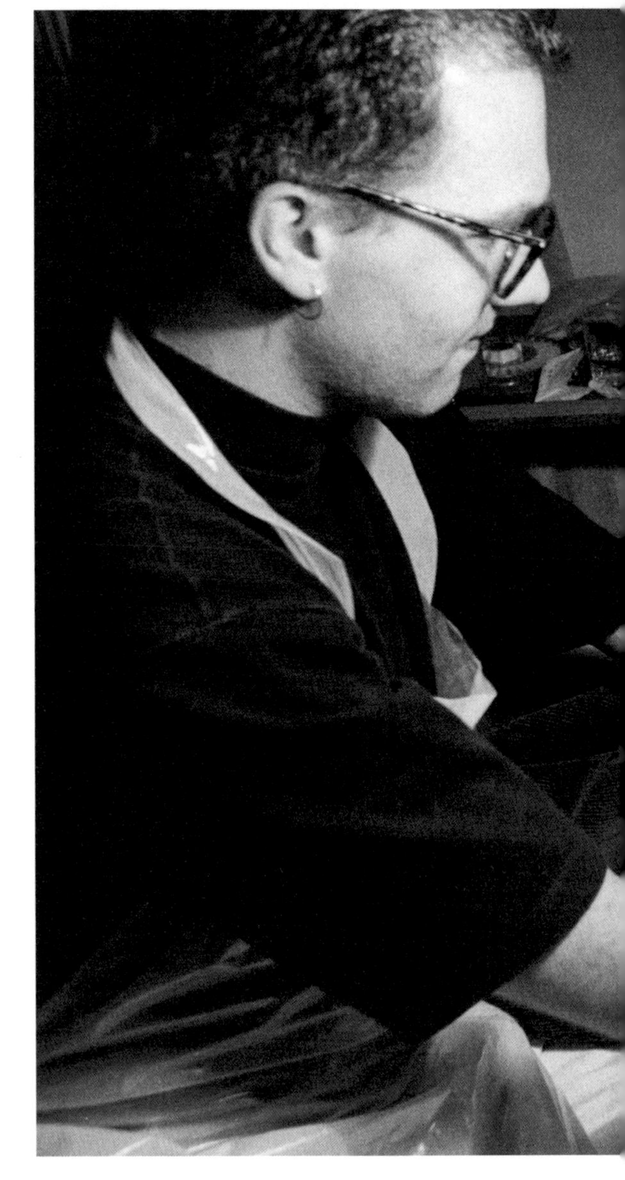

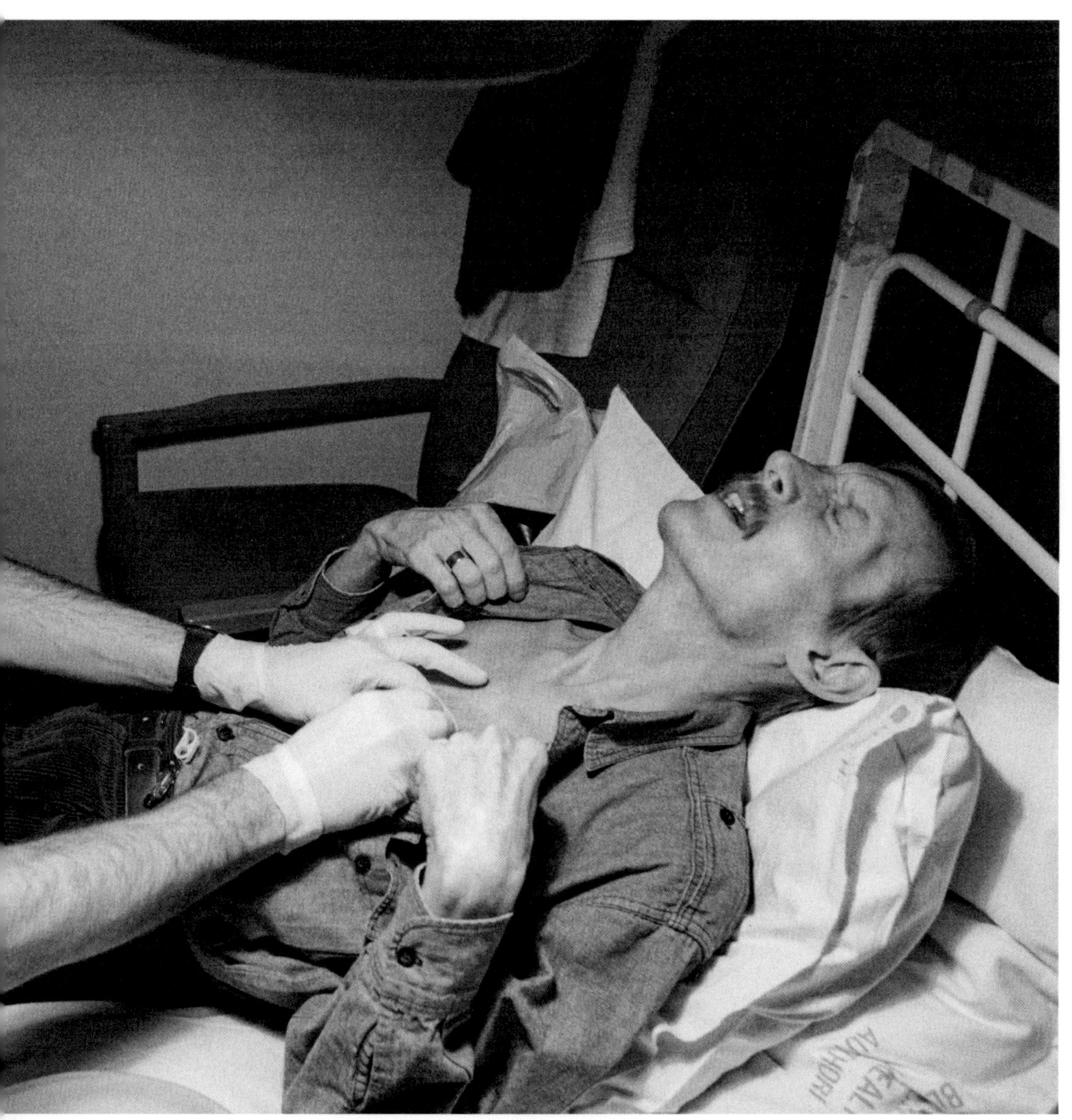

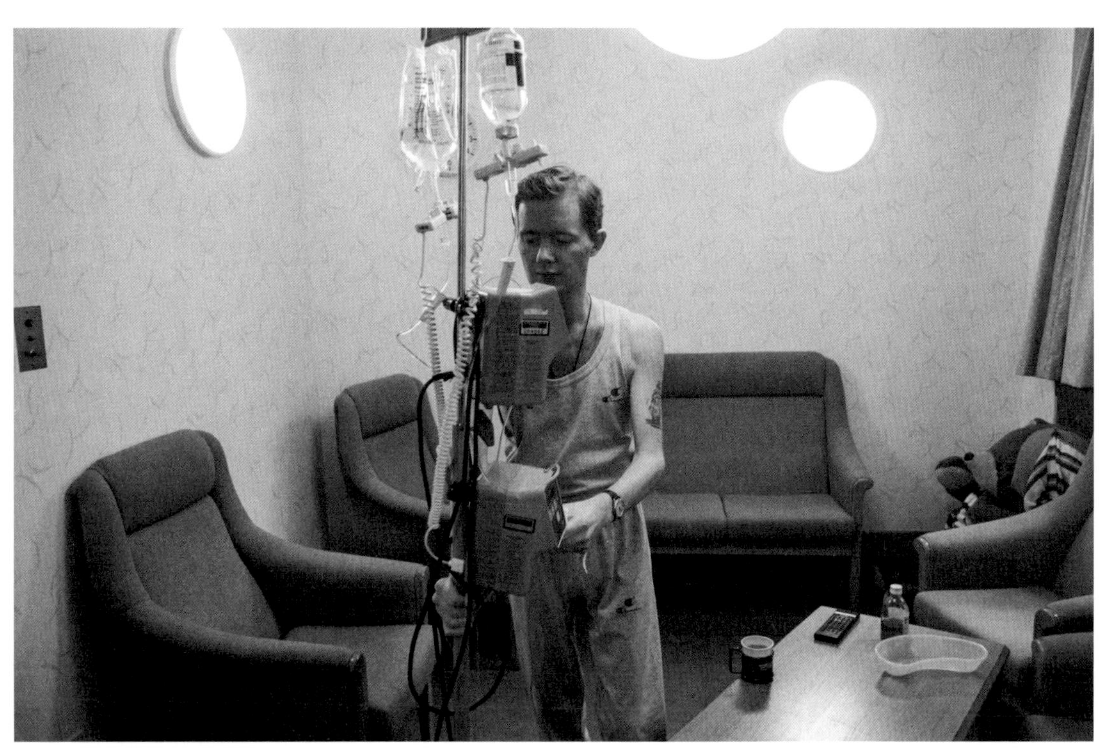

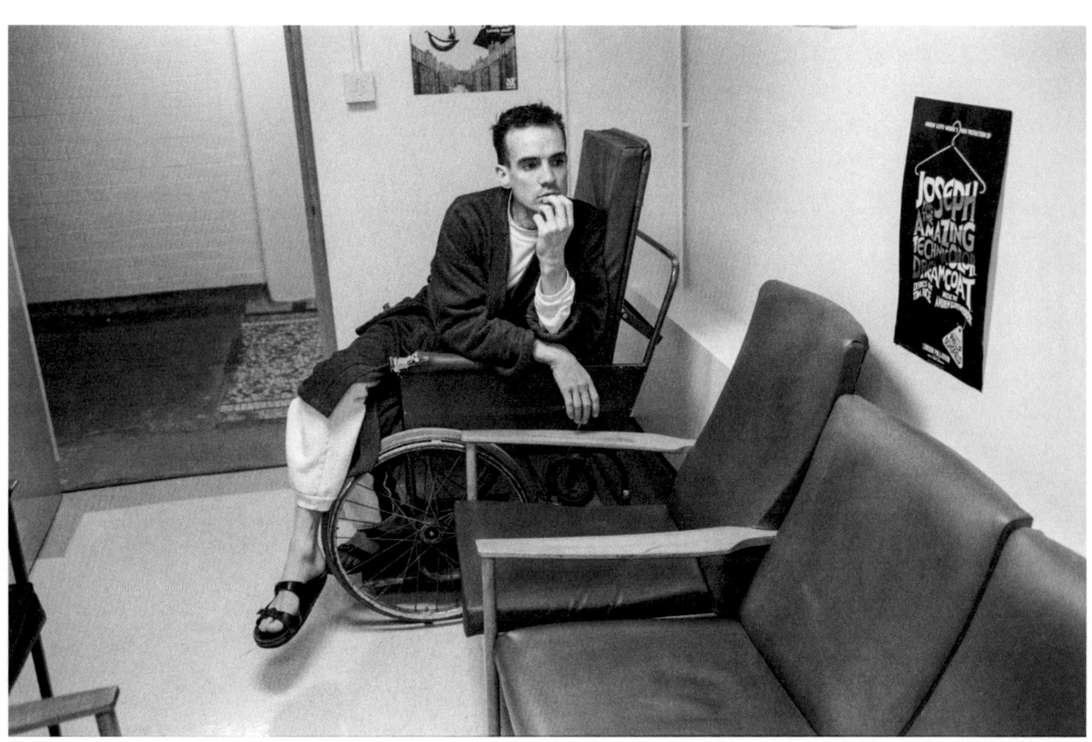
ANDREW LLOYD WEBBER'S NEW PRODUCTION OF
JOSEPH
AND THE
AMAZING
TECHNICOLOR
DREAMCOAT
LYRICS BY
TIM RICE
MUSIC BY
ANDREW LLOYD WEBBER
LONDON PALLADIUM

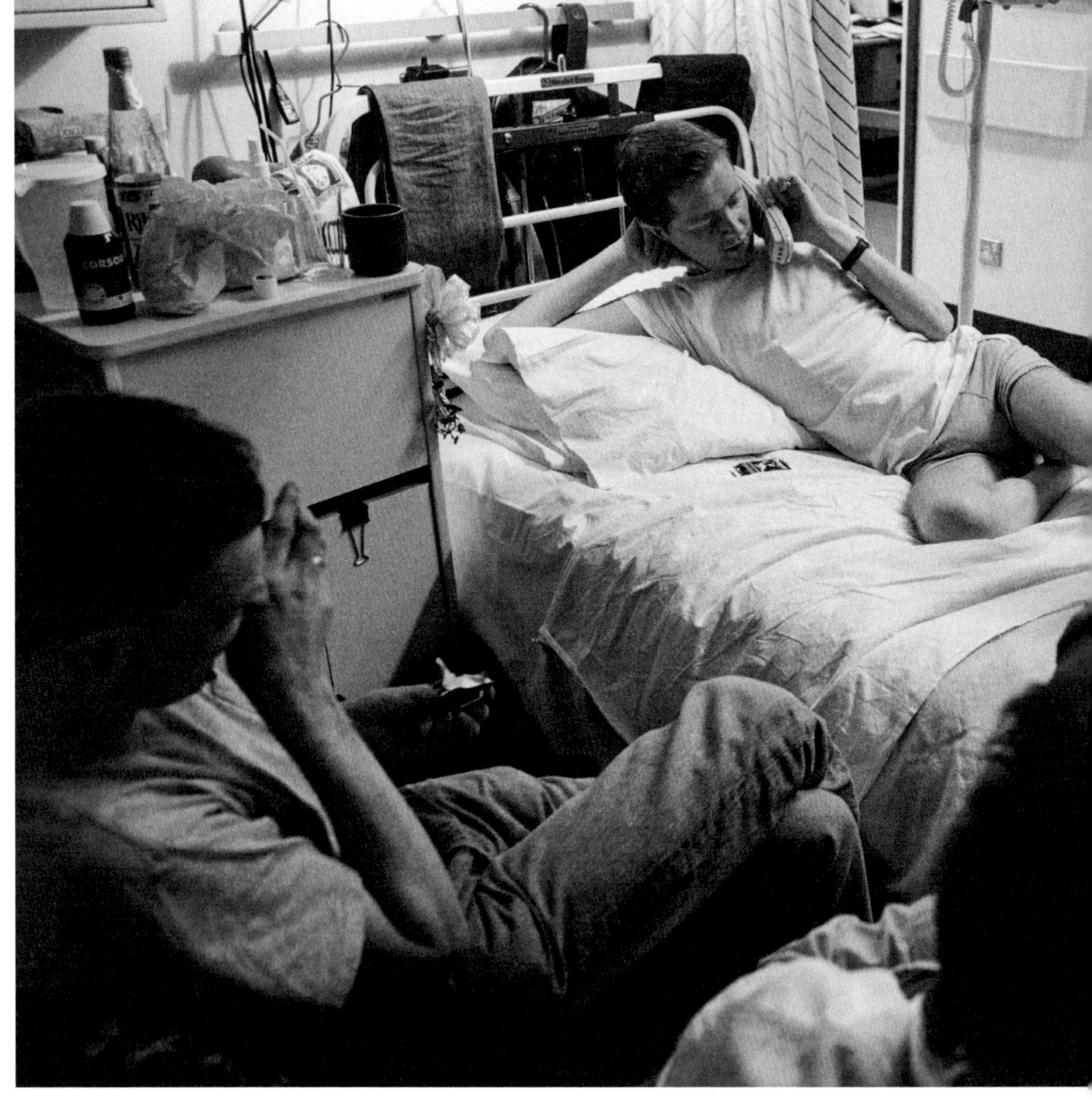

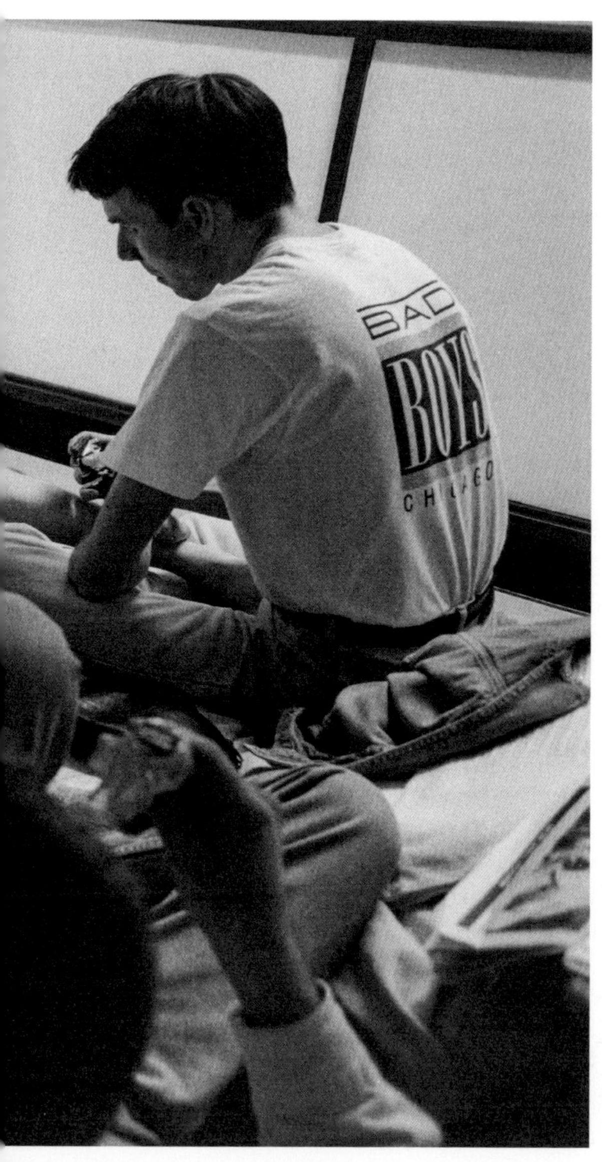

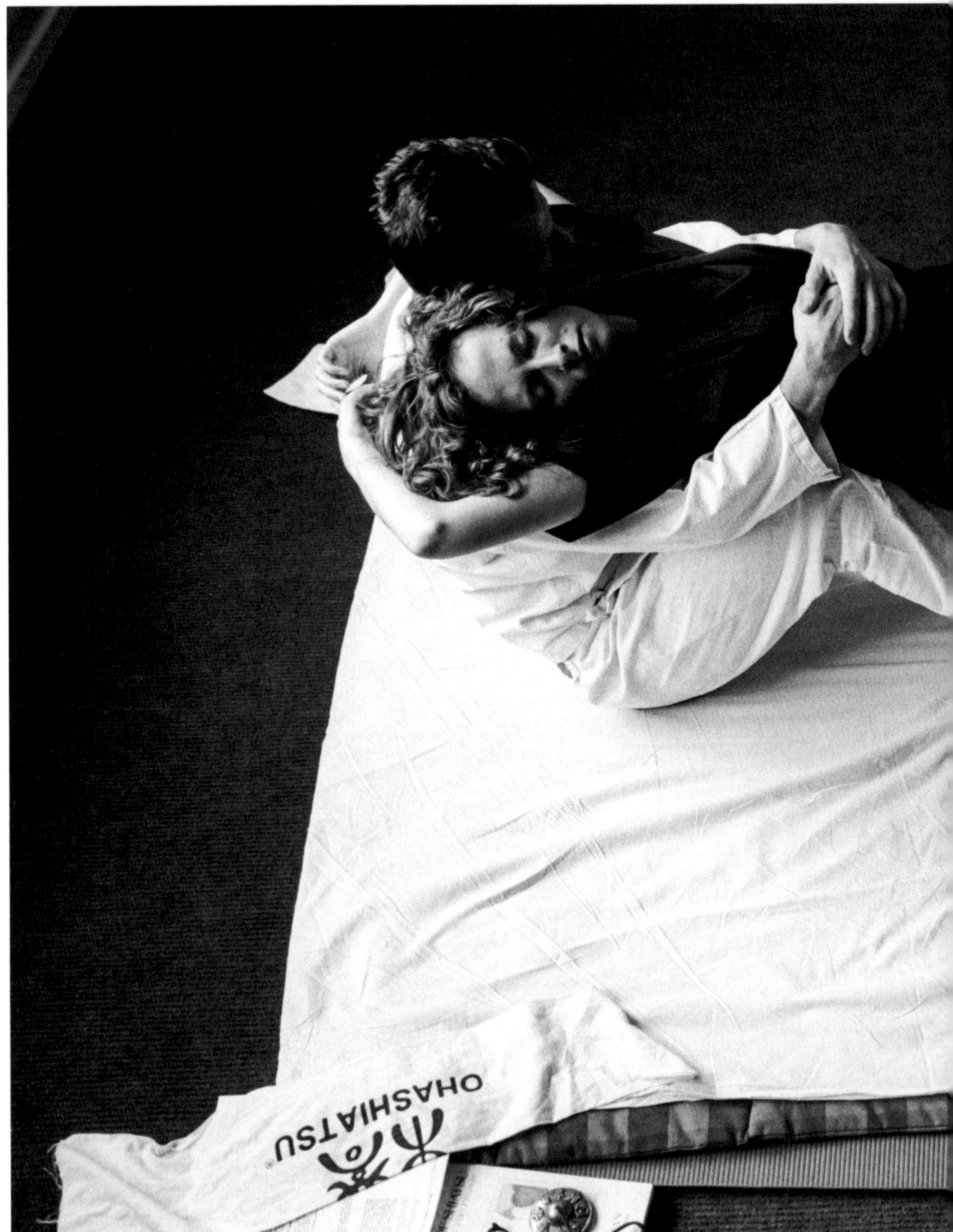
OHASHIATSU®

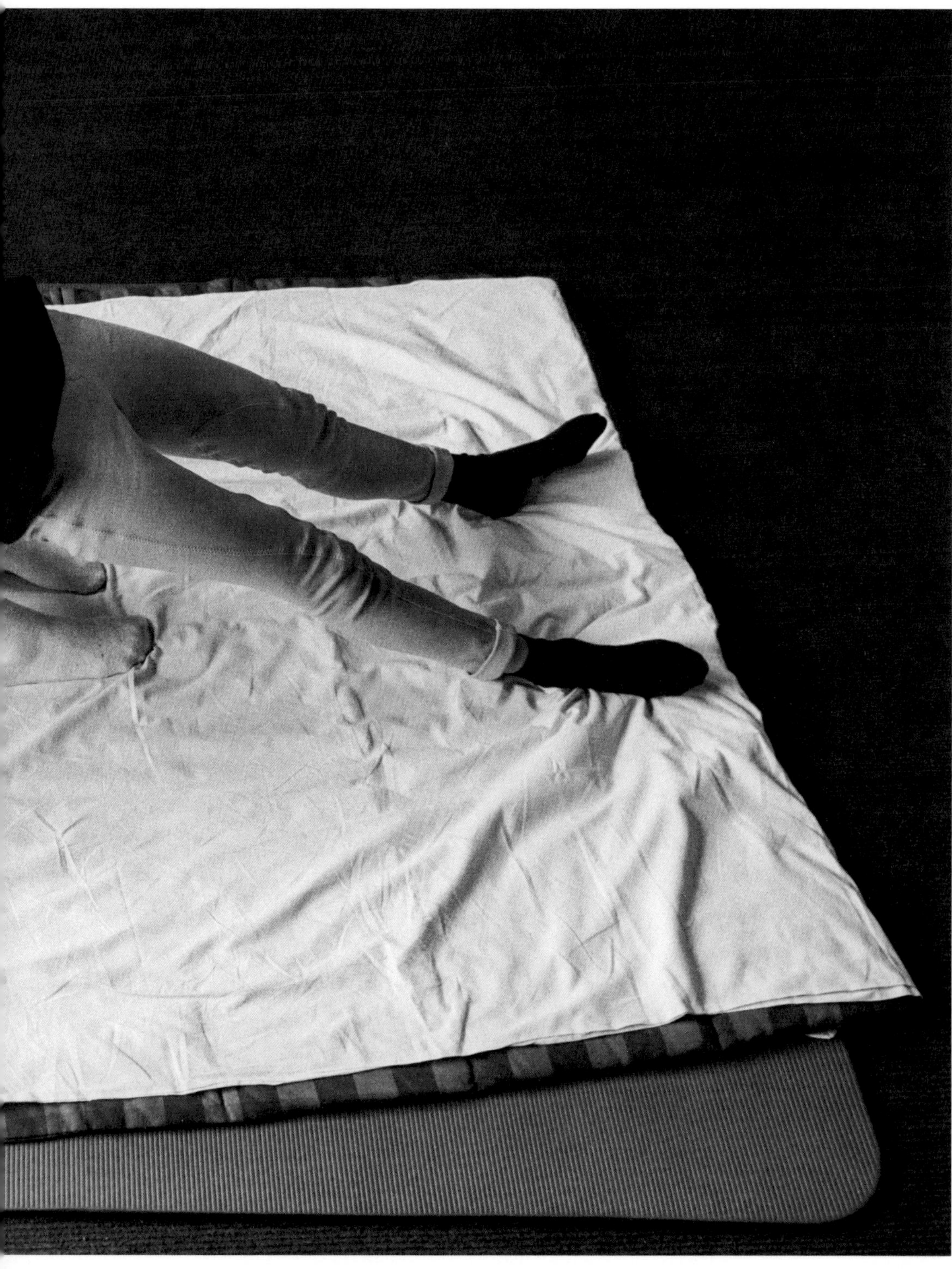

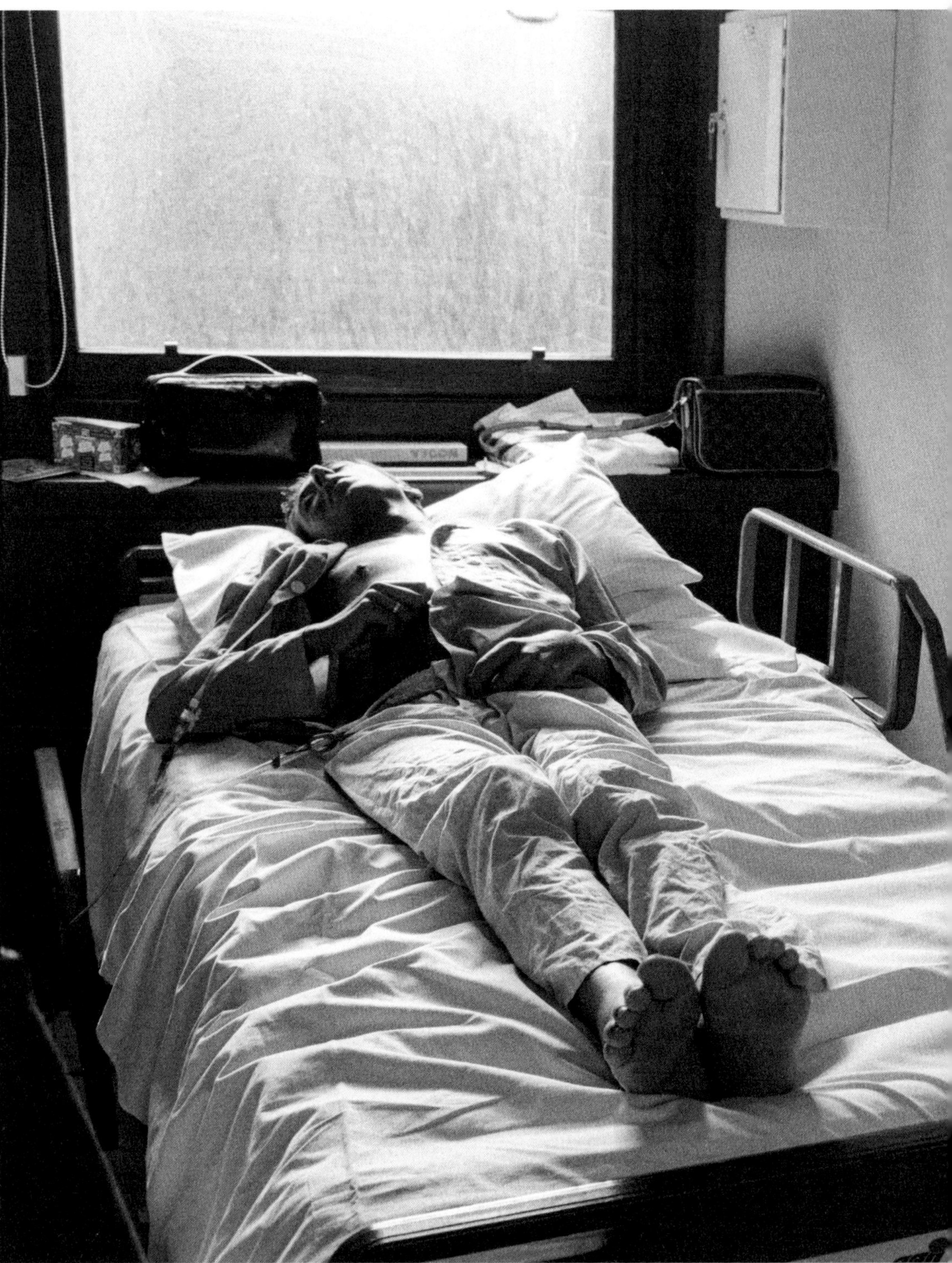

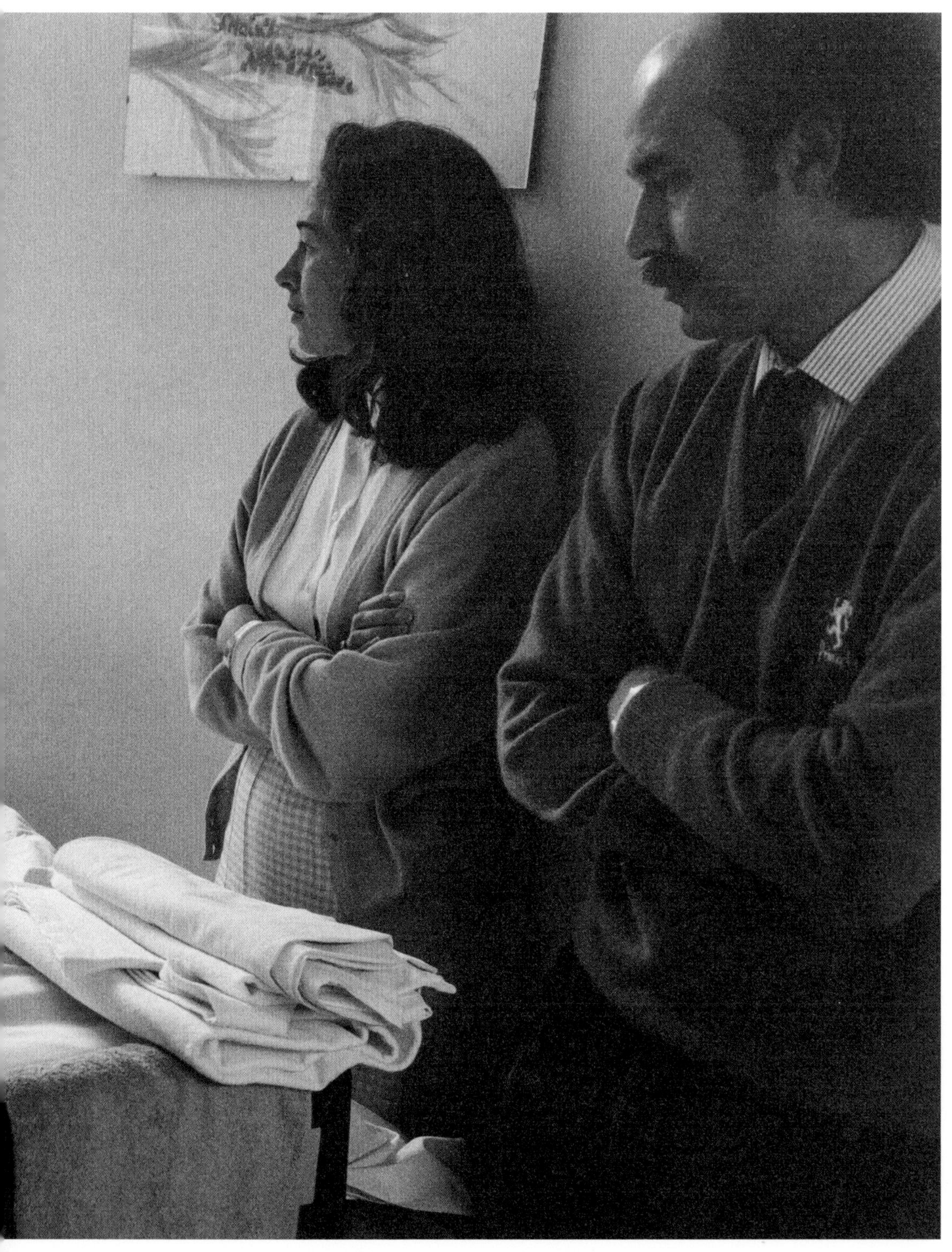

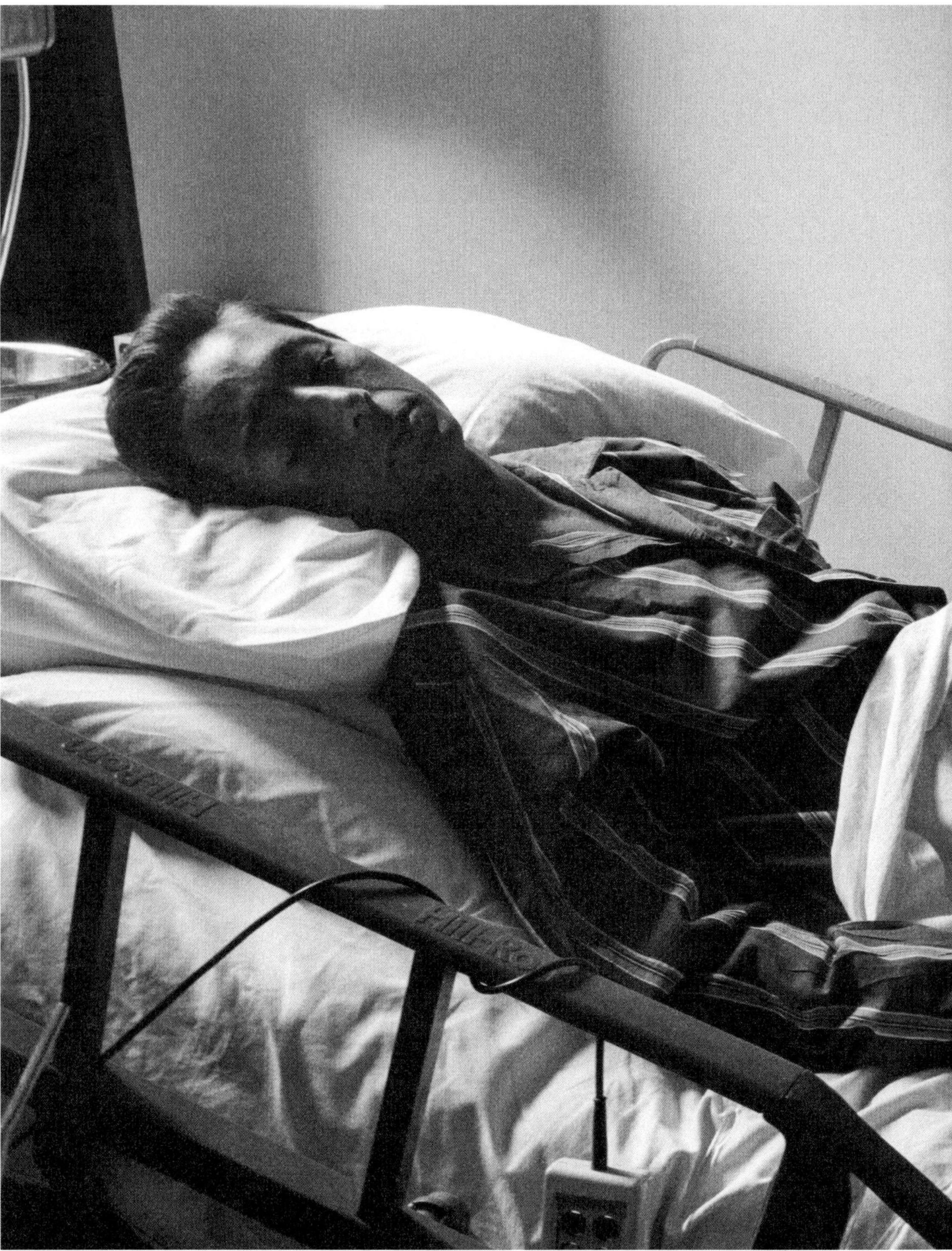

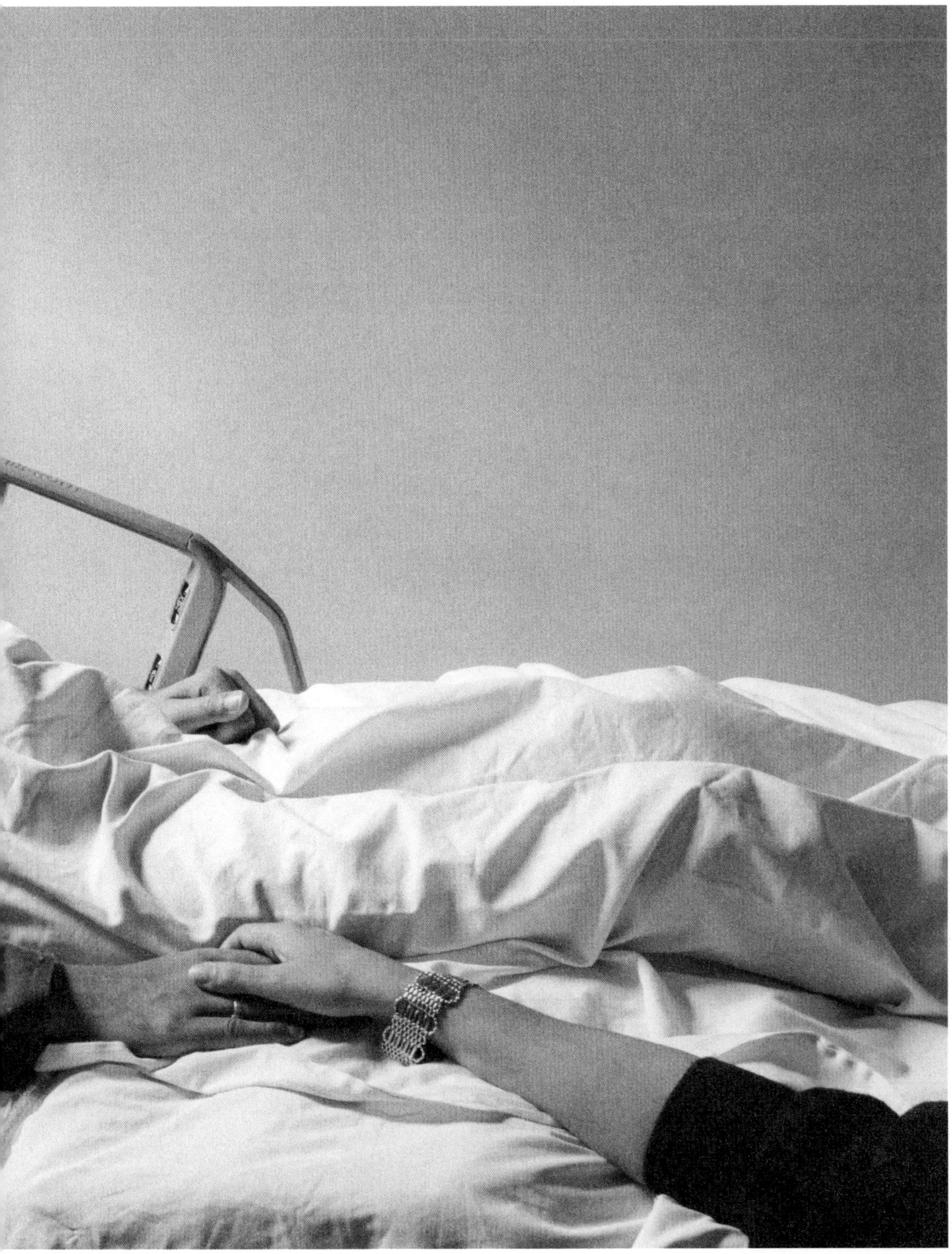

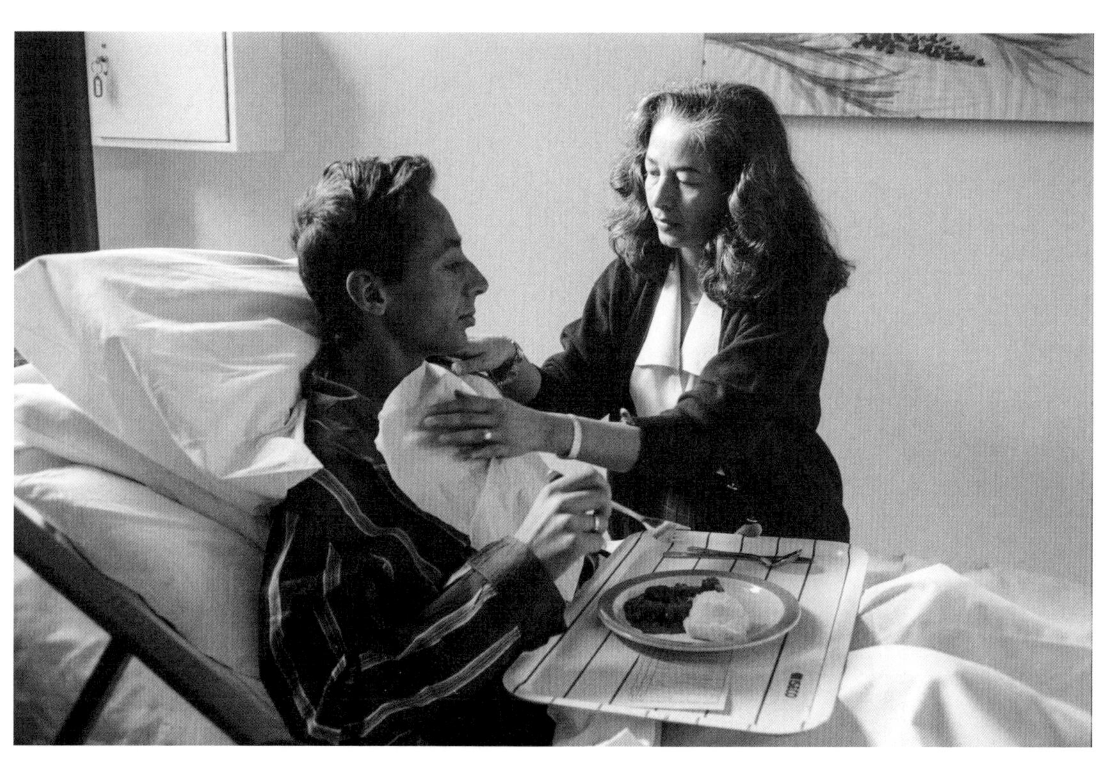

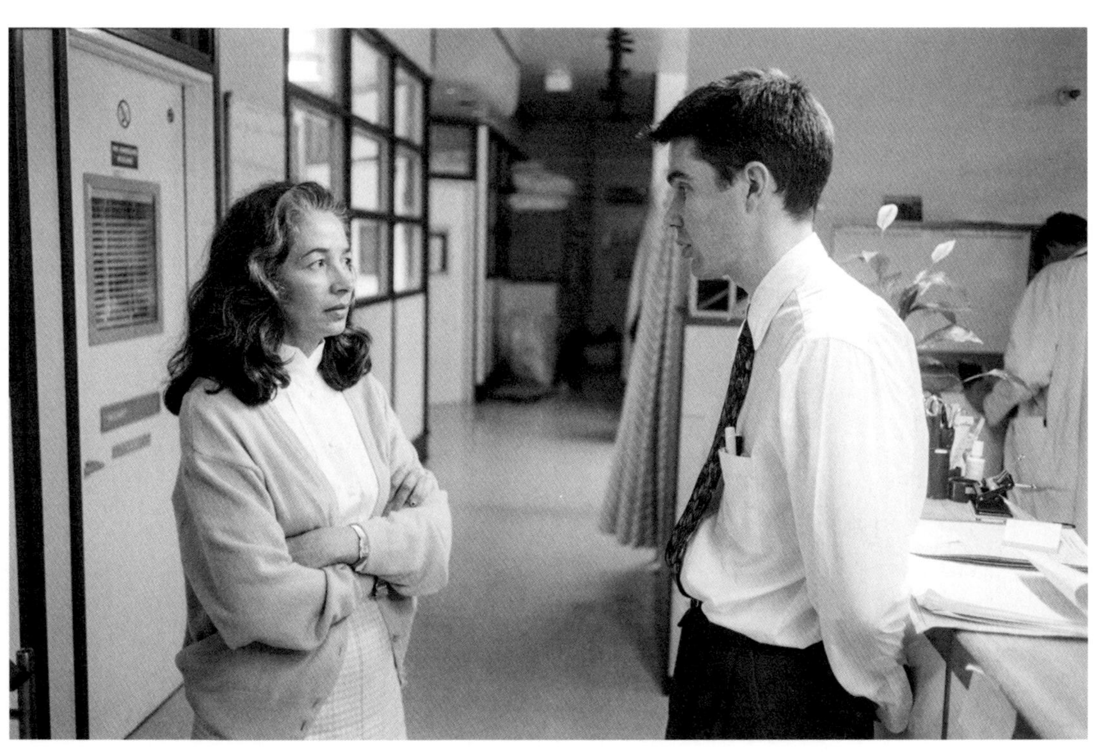

I first worked at The Middlesex Hospital as a medical registrar in 1989. Broderip ward had opened as the first HIV ward in the UK two years earlier (I remember watching Jacqui Elliott, the first ward sister, on the Terry Wogan chat show on TV shortly afterwards – it was national news). At first I worked in gastroenterology, and quickly found myself spending lots of time on Broderip seeing patients with swallowing problems or diarrhoea and weight loss, as nobody else in my department at the time was particularly interested in HIV. When I was on call at night as medical registrar for the hospital, most of my time was spent on Broderip and Charles Bell, because that is where the sickest patients were. The nursing staff on both wards were amazing – passionate, funny, warm, strong men and women who all chose to work in HIV, and were powerful advocates for their patients. The atmosphere on the wards was different from the rest of the hospital, and you felt it as you crossed the threshold walking onto Broderip. The patients were often really interesting – from different walks of life, but many writers, painters, actors and creative people – I remember a comment that somebody made that if only all the patients weren't so ill, they could put on a brilliant opera or make an amazing film.

I later became the ward registrar on Broderip and Charles Bell wards from August 1992 for 14 months. During that time I exclusively worked on the inpatient wards – there were 12 beds on Broderip, and a total of 15 on Charles Bell (this ward opened several years after Broderip), most of which were full nearly all of the time with people with advanced HIV. Cytomegalovirus retinitis (causing loss of vision) affected dozens of people, who had to learn to administer their own intravenous medication at home every day to avoid progressive loss of vision. They would be admitted, we would treat them for an infection or some other complication of HIV and they would go home, only to return perhaps a few months later with something else; the pattern repeated until they died. Sometimes they never went home in the first place. Virtually everyone I looked after during that period has died.

In September 1993, I left the Middlesex to work in the HIV unit at St. Mary's. Although the problems that my patients at St. Mary's had were the same, the work was outpatient based and far less intense, and it was only then that I realised how much of a toll the previous year or so had taken on me. Just a few years later, effective antiretroviral therapy became available, and suddenly we could stop people getting sick and dying, which was indescribably amazing. Being able to help people who were sometimes close to death get better and back to life was the most magical thing, made all the more so by my earlier experiences. I still look after some of the patients that I first met in the early 90s at St. Mary's, and I feel incredibly fortunate to have lived through the last 20-odd years with them.

**Dr Duncan Churchill,
registrar on Broderip and Charles Bell wards
1992 - 1993**

Do you remember Oscar Moore? Oscar Moore died of AIDS and I was one of the nurses caring for him on Broderip ward.

Oscar Moore used to write a column for the Weekend Guardian about living with AIDS from 1994 until his death in 1996. These articles were published in 1996 in a book entitled PWA Looking AIDS in the face by Picador. At the time I thought he continued to do for AIDS what Princess Diana had done when she visited the HIV/AIDS unit at the Middlessex Hospital. Her famous handshake with an "AIDS' patient" aimed at normalising the illness and ensured AIDS became an issue for all.

Early on in Oscar Moore's illness I had some honest and thought provoking conversations with him. I always felt that Oscar was open to looking at life deeply. He was not only interested in social niceties. 18 months later he came to the ward because he could not see after an eye operation. He felt he could not cope independently. He stayed for 3 days just to be looked after and cared for. There was a significant loss of independence. This forced a new humility. I think he was scared and it made me frightened for him. It was like a foreboding.

When Oscar came back in the summer of
1996, he deteriorated quickly and drifted in and
out of consciousness. I looked after him a lot then.
I remember washing him, listening to him cursing
me, the loss of control, the end. I looked at a
changed man. Yet every day I tried to convey to
him that even this end was okay. There were no
expectations of him or of the rest of his life. His
worth was unchanged by the circumstances of his
debilitating illness.

I was on night duty the night Oscar Moore
died. He died very quietly, and I thought of the
words so often used: "he just slipped away". That
is how it was.

I went to his funeral and the farewell was hard.
There were many people, some of whom I had met
in the preceding years. I realised that I would not
see them again, but that we had all been touched
by Oscar's life. As a friend said: his journey is over,
yet he continues to shape mine.

**Barbara Von Barsewisch,
nurse on the Broderip ward,
1993 - 1994**

It was early in my career and definitely the highlight. We ran on a heady mixture of adrenalin and emotions of compassion, grief, sadness and love. We were finding things out every day. There was a fear of the unknown and the known was grim.

Just before my time at James Pringle House the doctors and health advisors were telling people following a HIV test, "You have the anti-bodies – you should be all right". Soon after people had to be recalled and told, "It is bad news," in fact, "Very bad news".

At first glance this was a medical problem, a challenge to the specialisms of immunology, virology, genito-urinary medicine, internal medicine, respiratory medicine, etc., but the psychological impact of what was unfolding was soon evident. Uncertainty, fear, anxiety, dealing with stigma, guilt, anger, loss and grief. There wasn't a 'Psychology' to deal with this, and Health Psychology was at its infancy. In the UK, David Miller and John Green emerged as pioneers who were in the frontline facing this unfolding catastrophe. They, and a few others, lay the foundations for the psychological response that we were to follow. While they watched how things were unfolding across the pond, they didn't copy the US responses but formulated a British approach. The WHO wanted someone to lead the global response and David Miller was seconded from the Middlesex Hospital to the WHO in Geneva, leaving a considerable gap at home.

I was working in the Addictions service, my first job as a clinical psychologist, in what was then Camden and Islington Health Authority. The psychology department spanned the Middlesex and University College Hospital as well as primary care and community services. I was recruited by David Miller, I can't remember the exact circumstances it was either in a pub or at a party, and I recall he was very persuasive. When I confessed to my ignorance of health psychology, let alone aspect of GU medicine, David dismissed this as irrelevant. My initial anxiety was soon dissipated by the warmth of the welcome by the team of health advisors led by Dorothy who soon became my family. Heather, Jan, Jane, Rene, Andrew, Sarah, joined by Alison, Deepti and

Debbie, they all have a special place in my heart. I can look back and say with honesty that together with the staff at Broderip and Charles Bell these were the nicest people I have ever worked with. The cosy warm and caring atmosphere, support for each other was unique. No doubt brought together because of the intensity of the challenges we were dealing with. It was immense, and looking back most of us gave beyond our capacities, I think the word "boundaries" in a psychological sense was not discovered by us back then. I think we identified with our patients and most of the time we were dealing with emotions that could not be easily contained. I know this was the same with the nursing team led by Jane and the medical team. I remember Tim Acton who was part of the psychology team at the beginning, after a long day and evening working with patients and families at Broderip, exhausted and saying "I really can't give any more". I remember during the early days when someone I worked with died, I would go to the chapel at the Middlesex Hospital and spend a few moments in contemplation. This practice was soon abandoned, as more and more patients started to die, and the workload would not allow for such luxuries. The inevitable result was burnout and when the triple retroviral treatments arrived, some of us had already left the field. Twenty-five years on memories of patients I worked with are as clear as yesterday, they were special and unforgettable and if they were not taken away so soon, they could have given the world so much. I feel very privileged to have been part of that tragic but very special time and place. It certainly taught me the meaning of caring.

Dr Shamil Wanigaratne
Clinical Psychologist, Middlesex Hospital
1989 - 1992

I worked on Charles Bell and Broderip wards
as a health adviser between 1989 and 1994.
In my almost 30 years in the NHS, this is the
time that stands out as the best of my career.
I've never worked in another environment that
was such a true collaboration between patients
and professionals. It was the days before really
effective treatments for HIV were available, and the
medical teams were at the cutting edge, constantly
researching and trying whatever they could to
combat the progress of the illness, and the patients
worked alongside them, and with all of us. We were
in it together. It did feel like being in battle with a
band of brothers and sisters, and we lost too many
in the course of that battle. I often think of them,
those that we lost, and their families and partners
who we got to know just as well. My role involved
advocating for patients to help meet social care
and housing needs, and supporting them and their
families to live with the illness and its progress,
and with the grieving process, through their time in
the hospital, both as inpatients and outpatients. I
feel so privileged to have had that time with them,
and I'll never forget them. The Middlesex was a
wonderful hospital and the ward staff were second
to none, this was the best of the NHS.

Heather Wilson, health adviser
Broderip and Charles Bell wards,
1989 - 1994

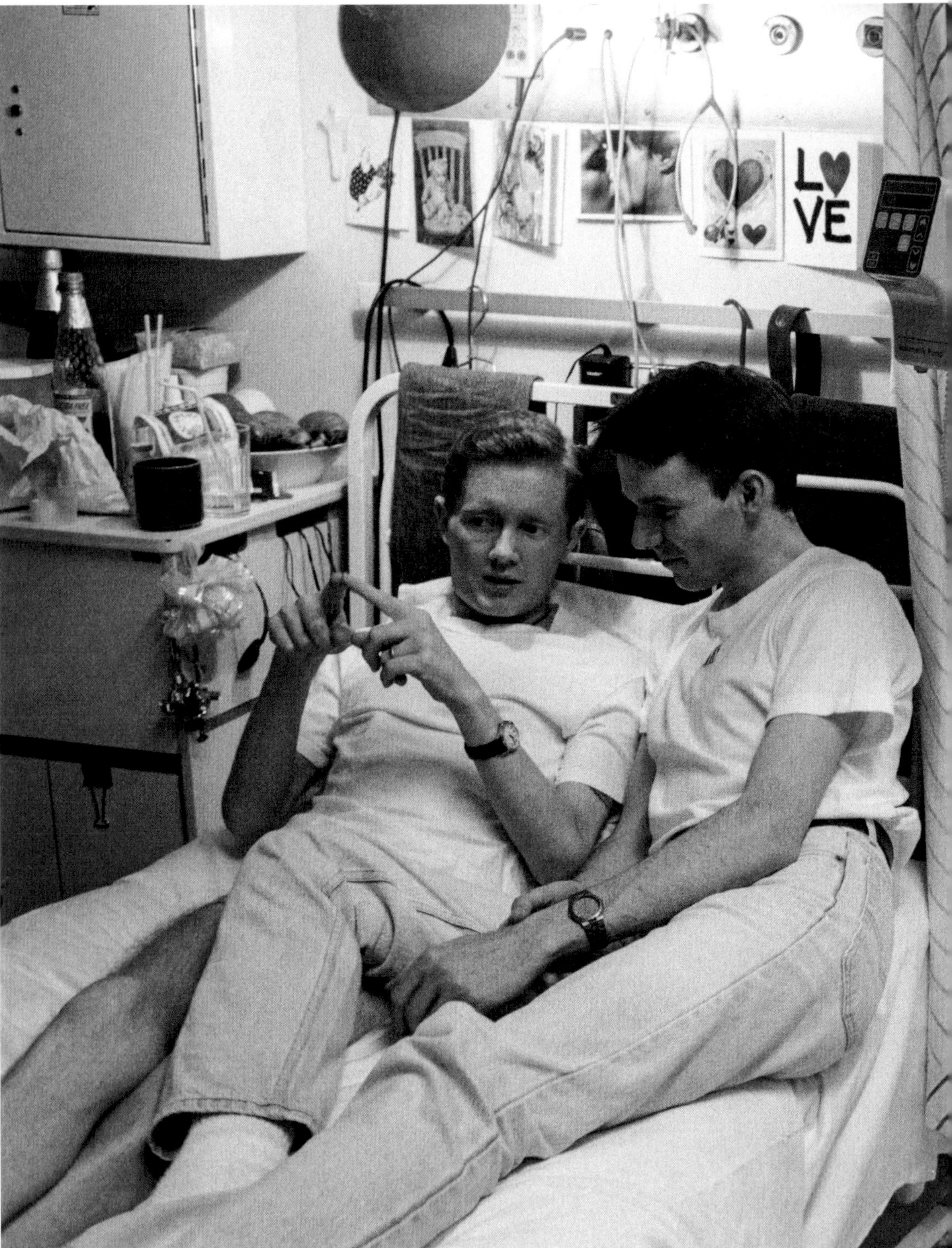

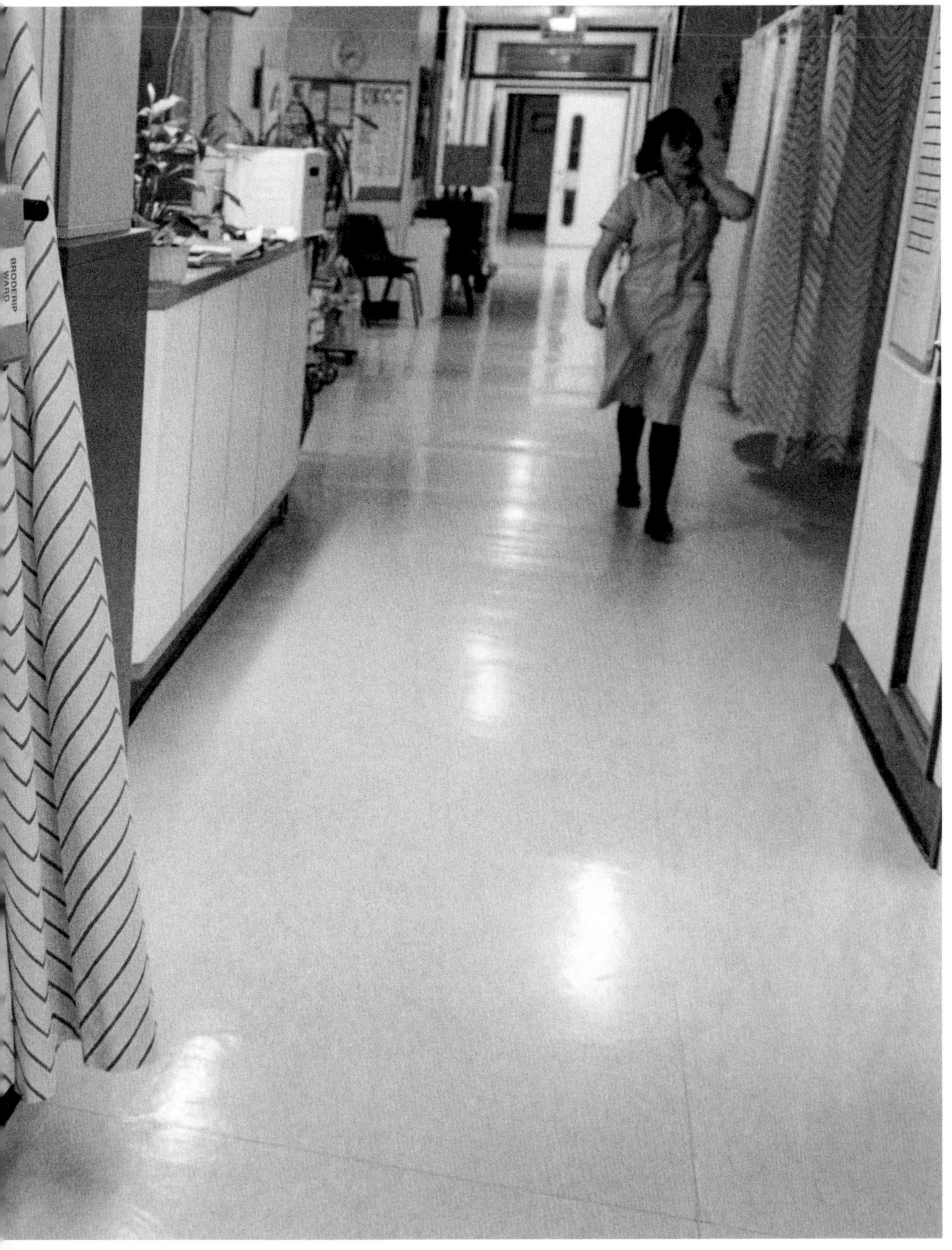
BRODERIP
WARD

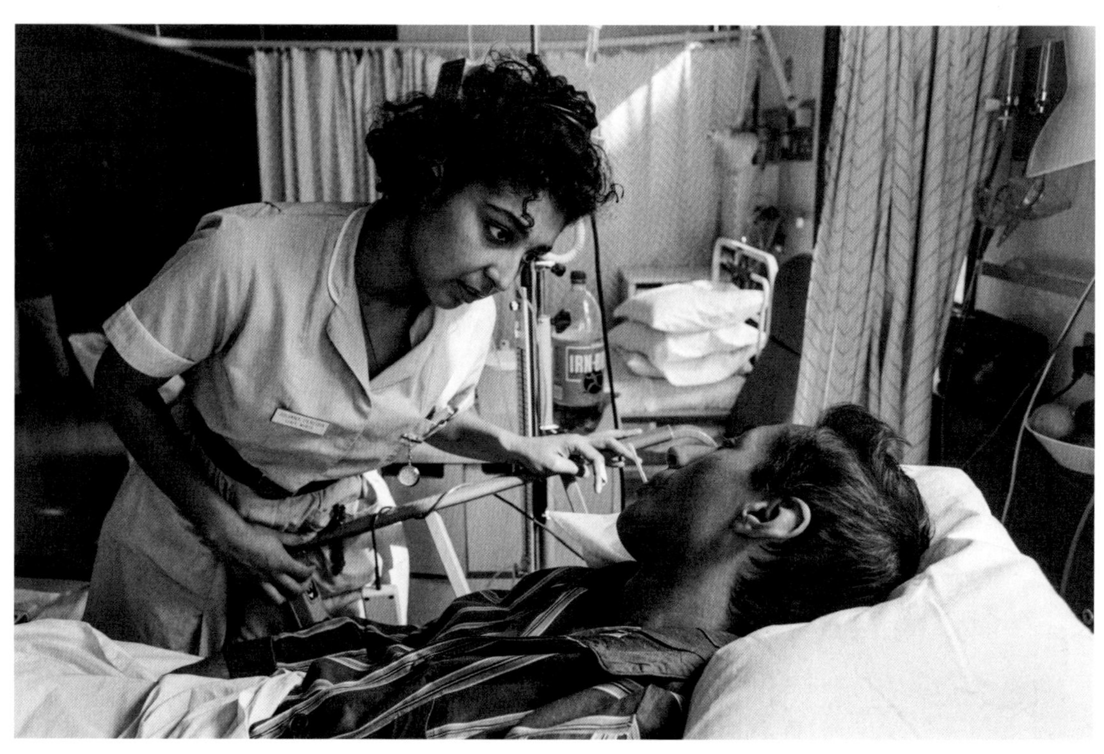

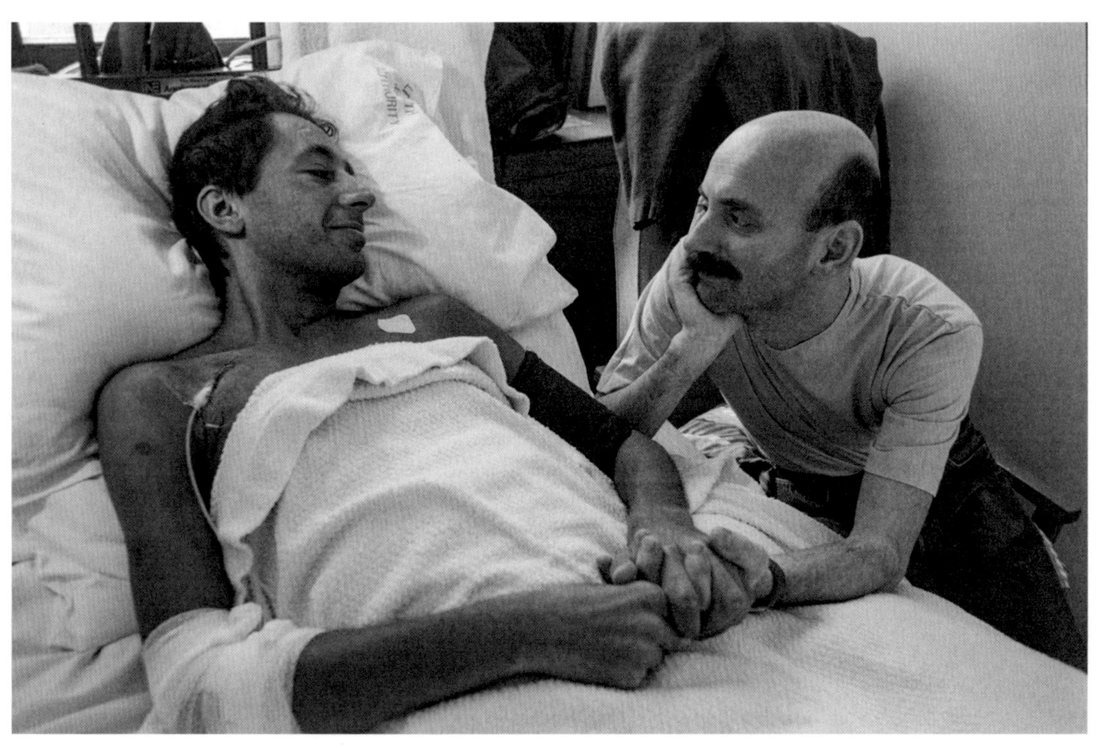

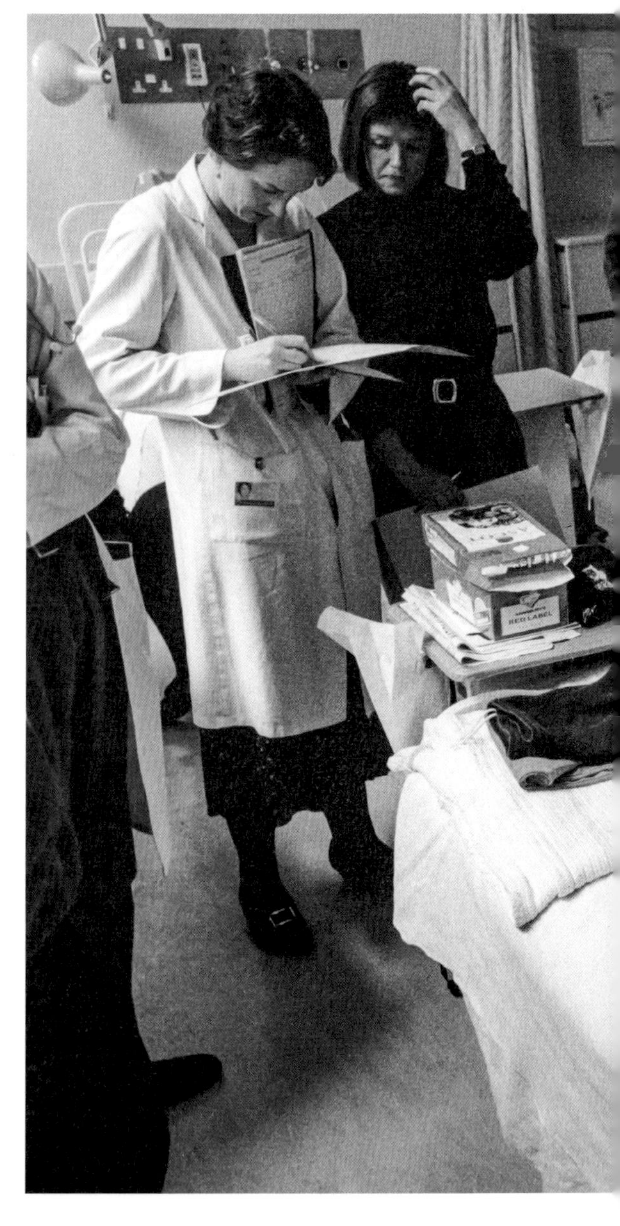

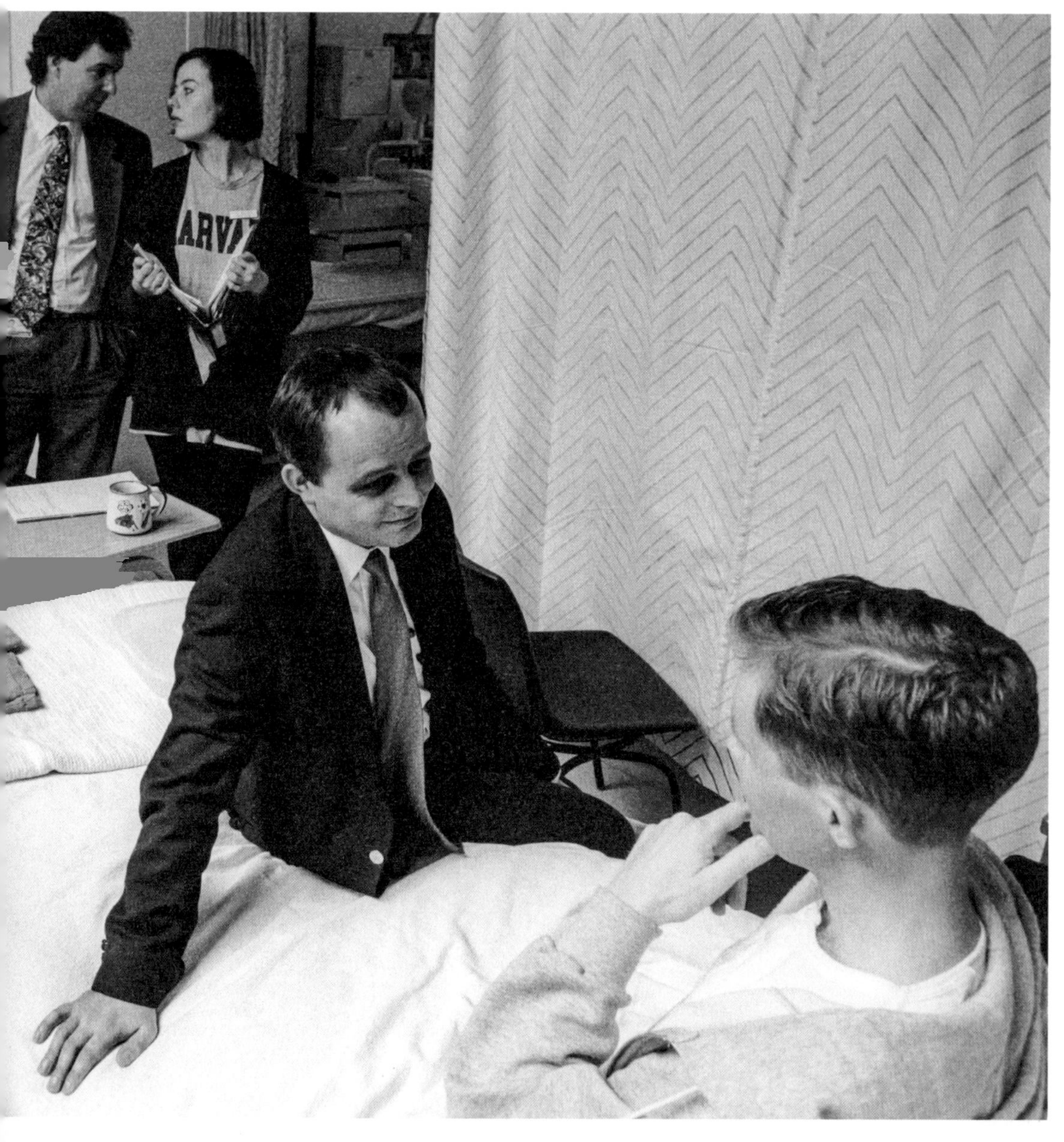

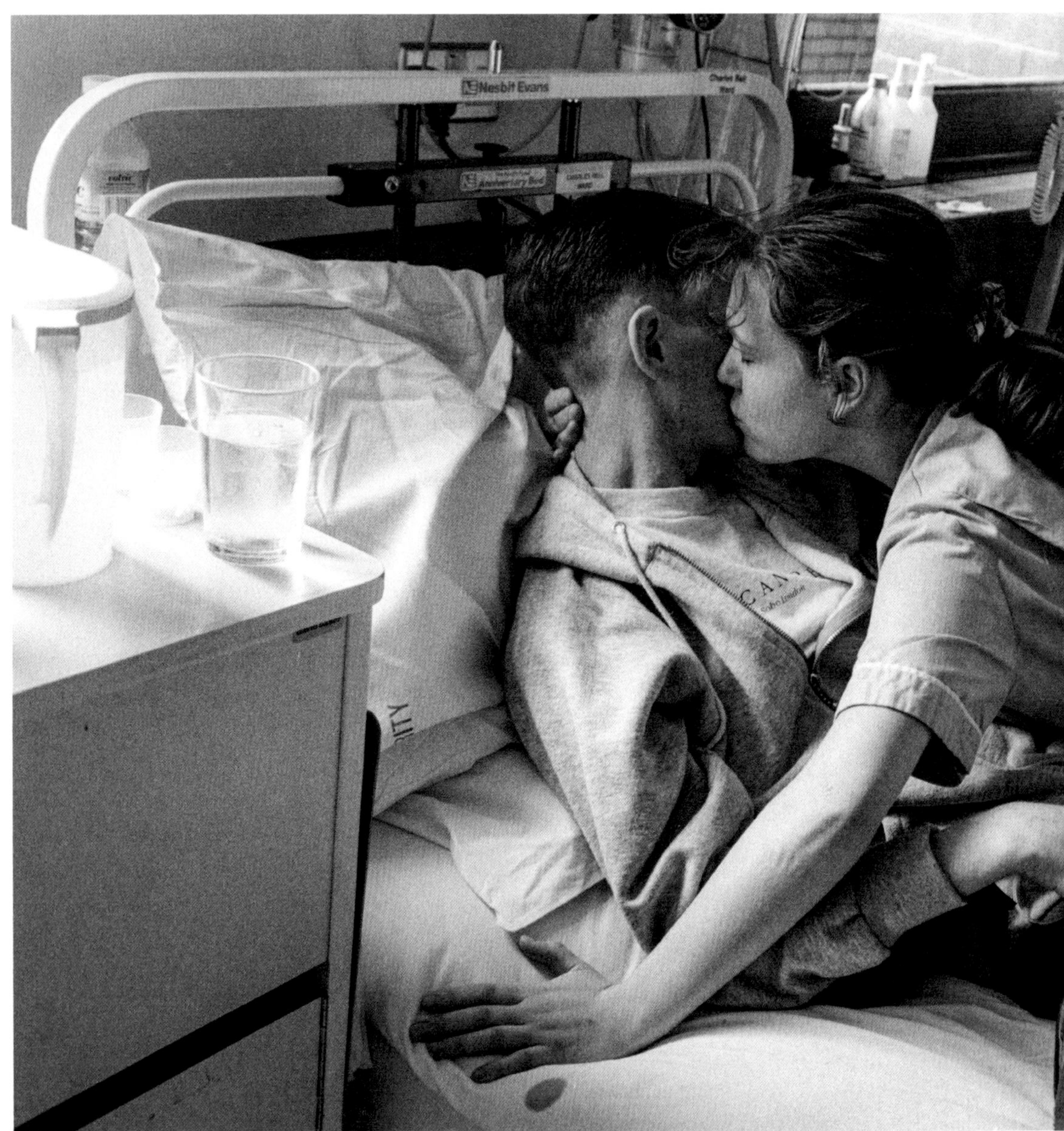

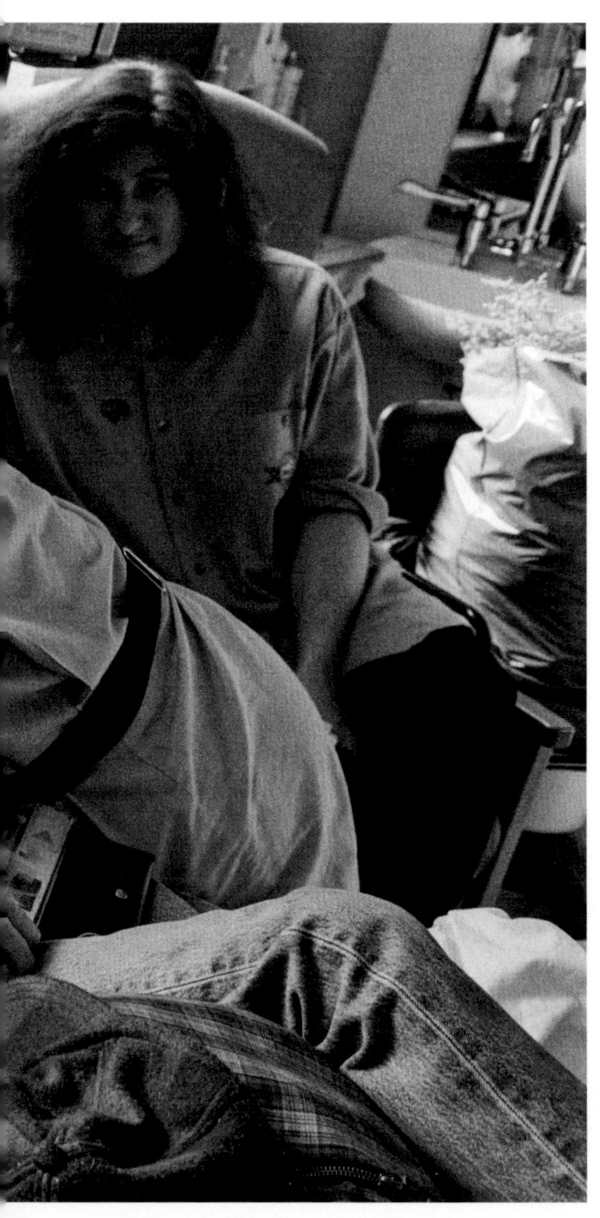

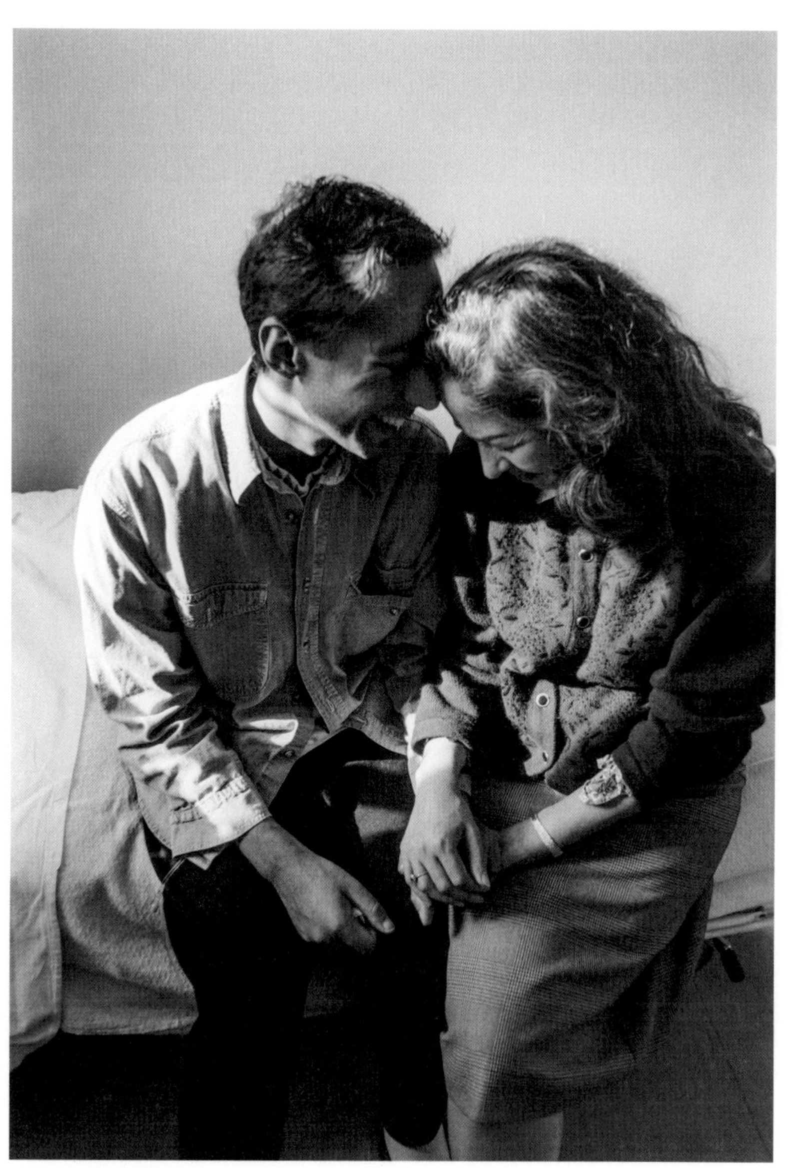

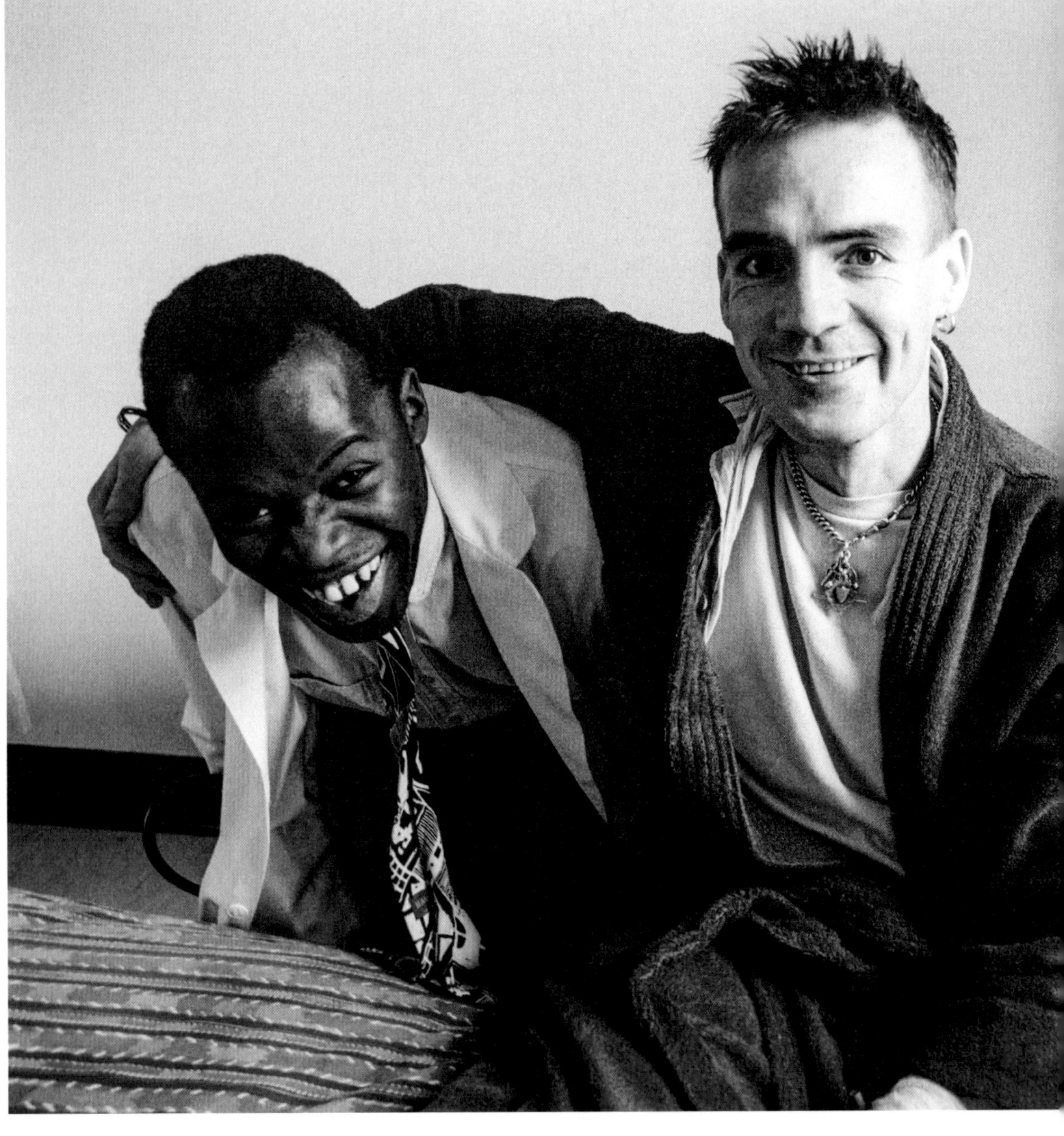

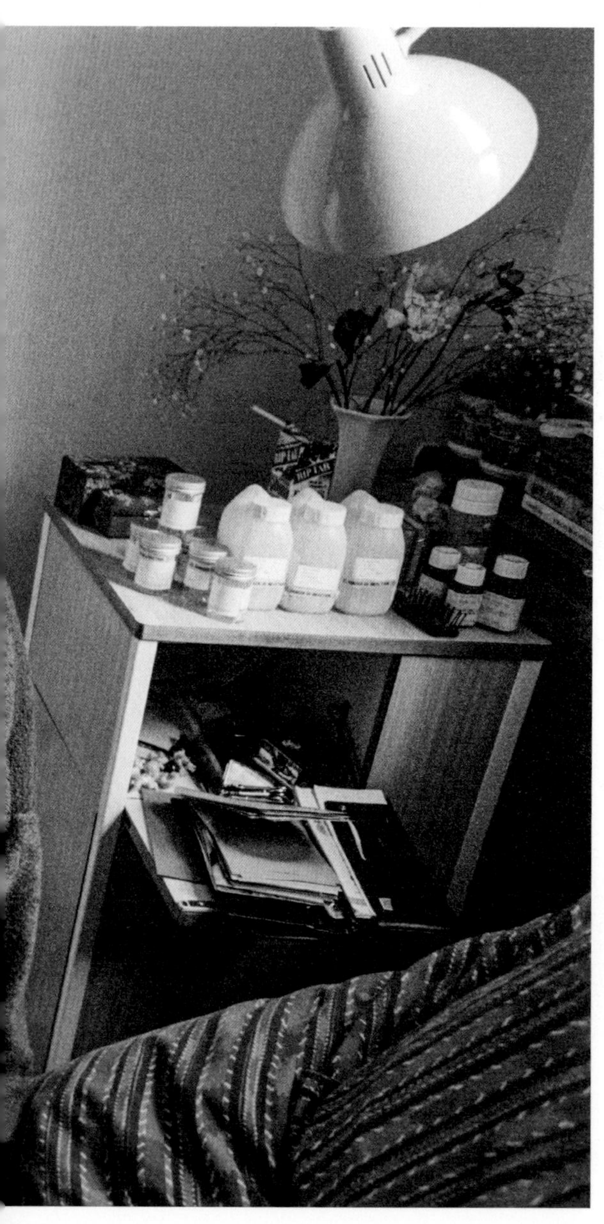

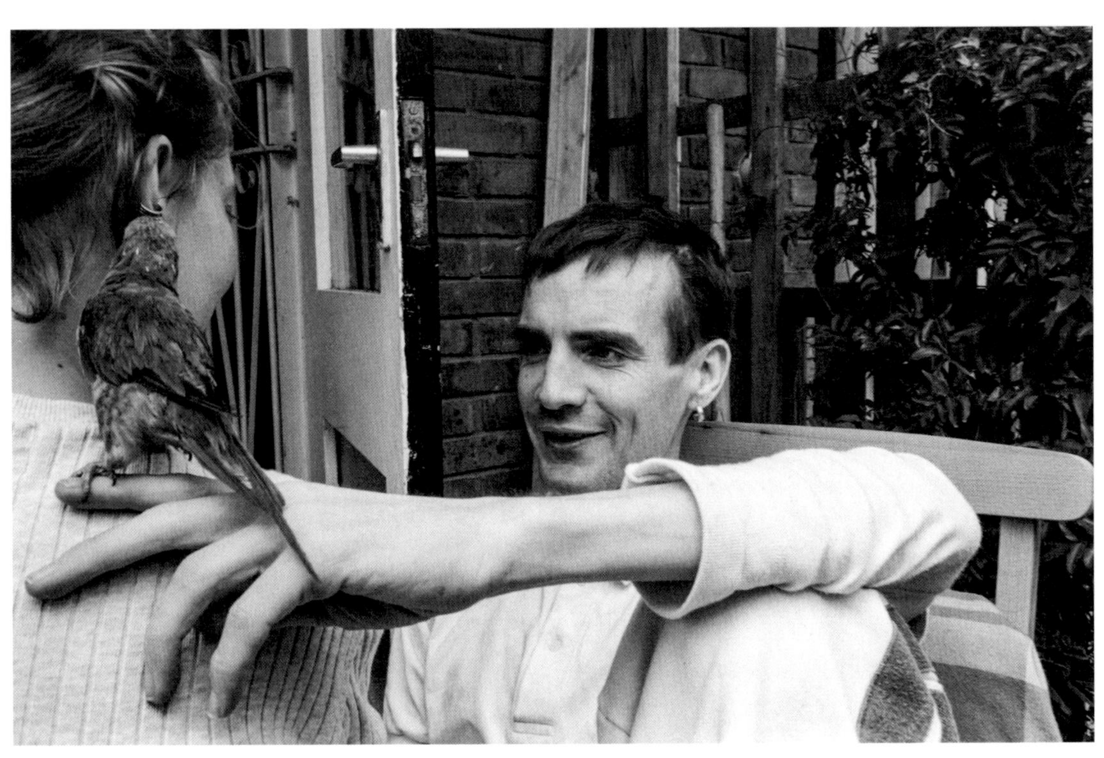

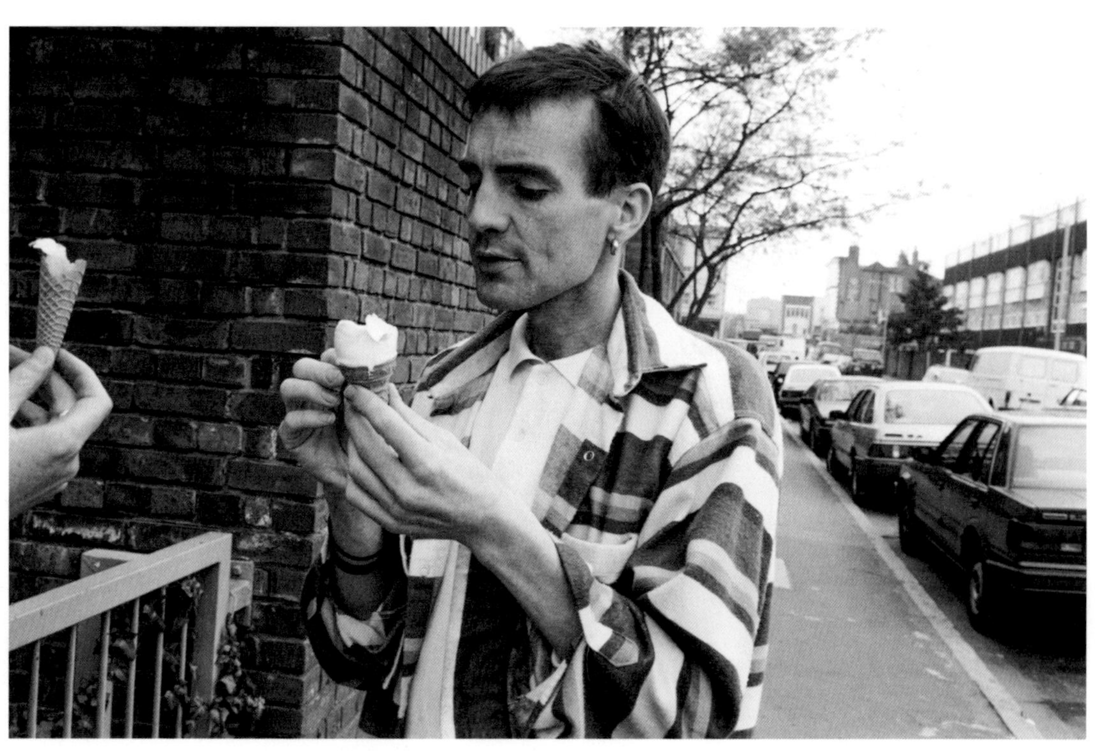

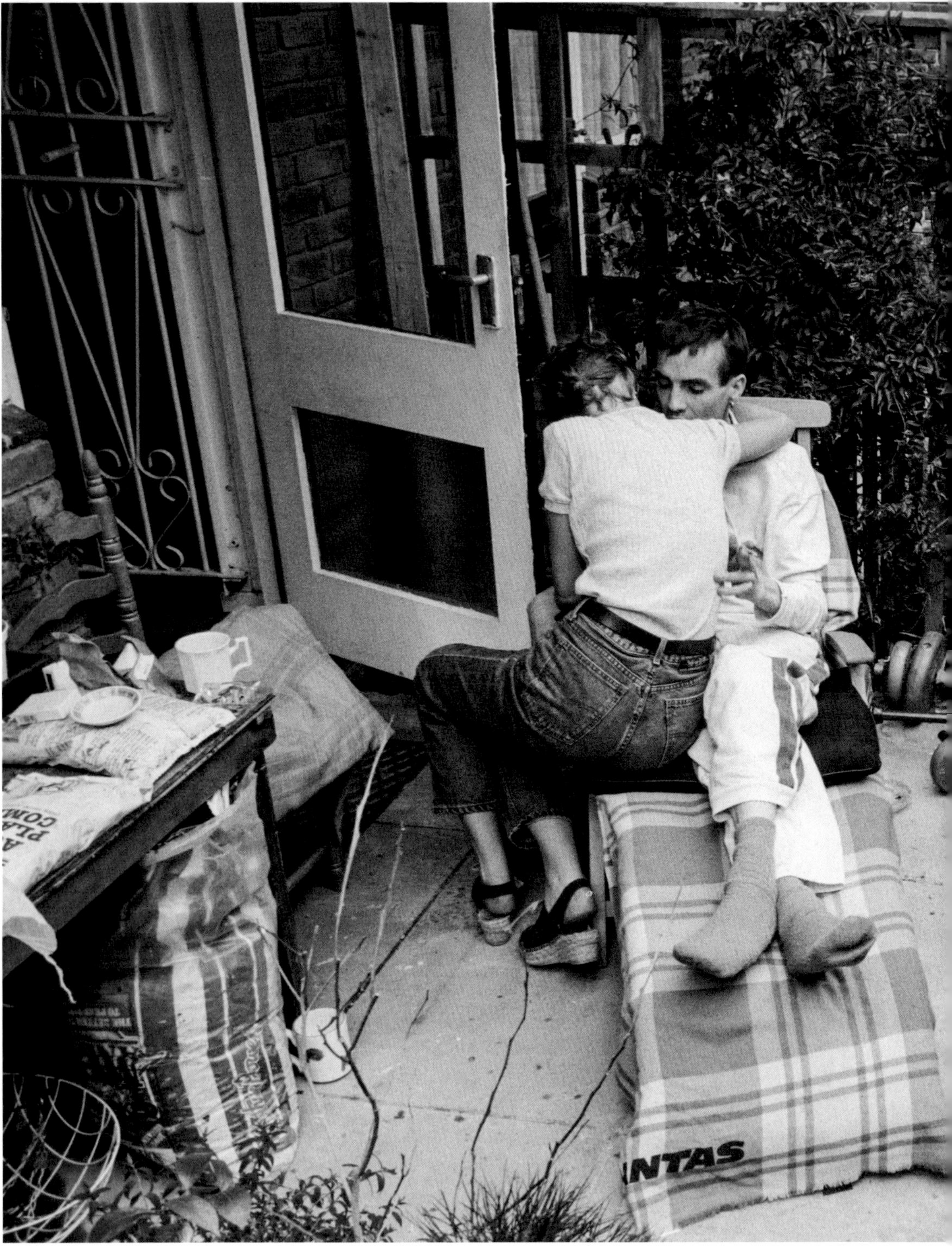
NTAS

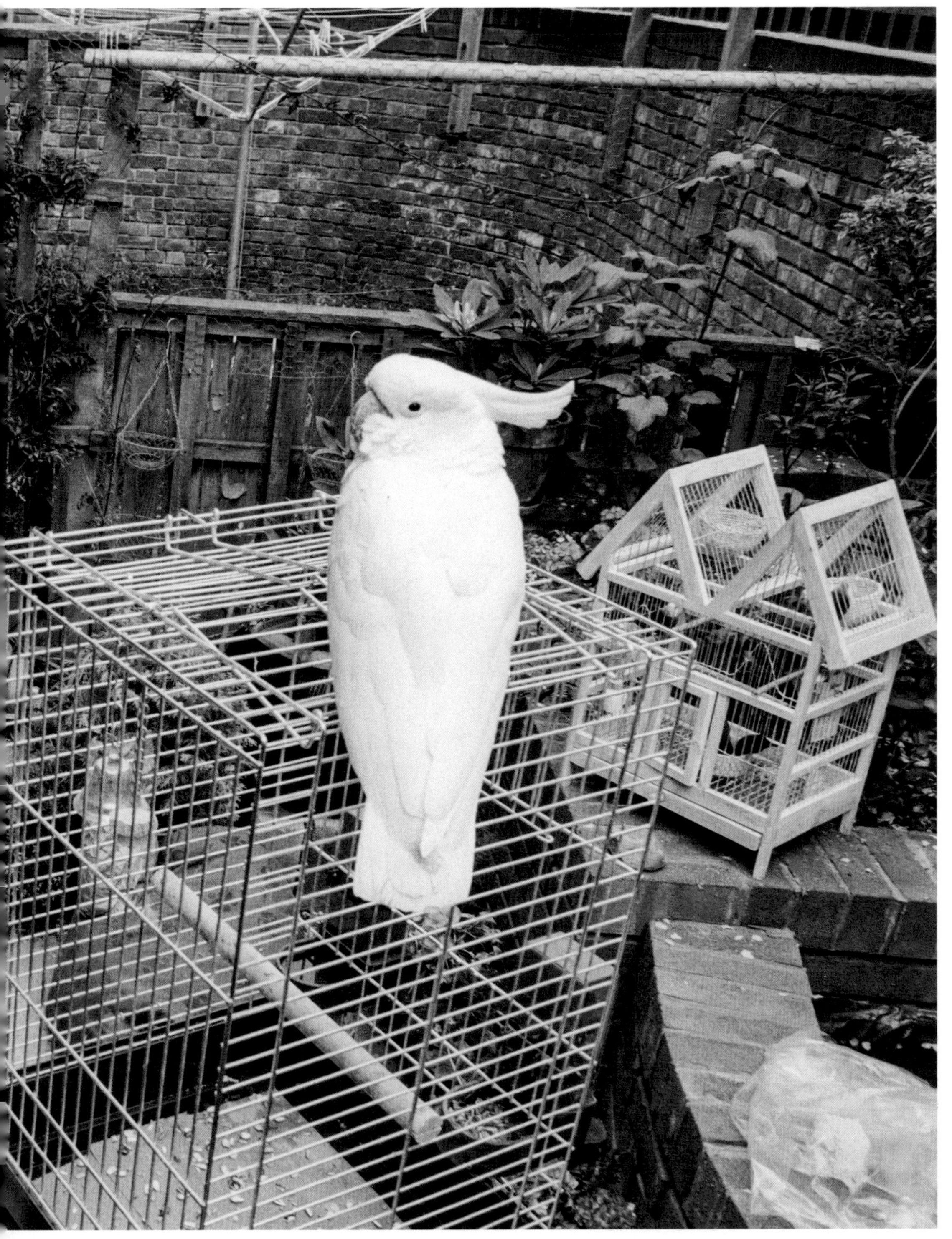

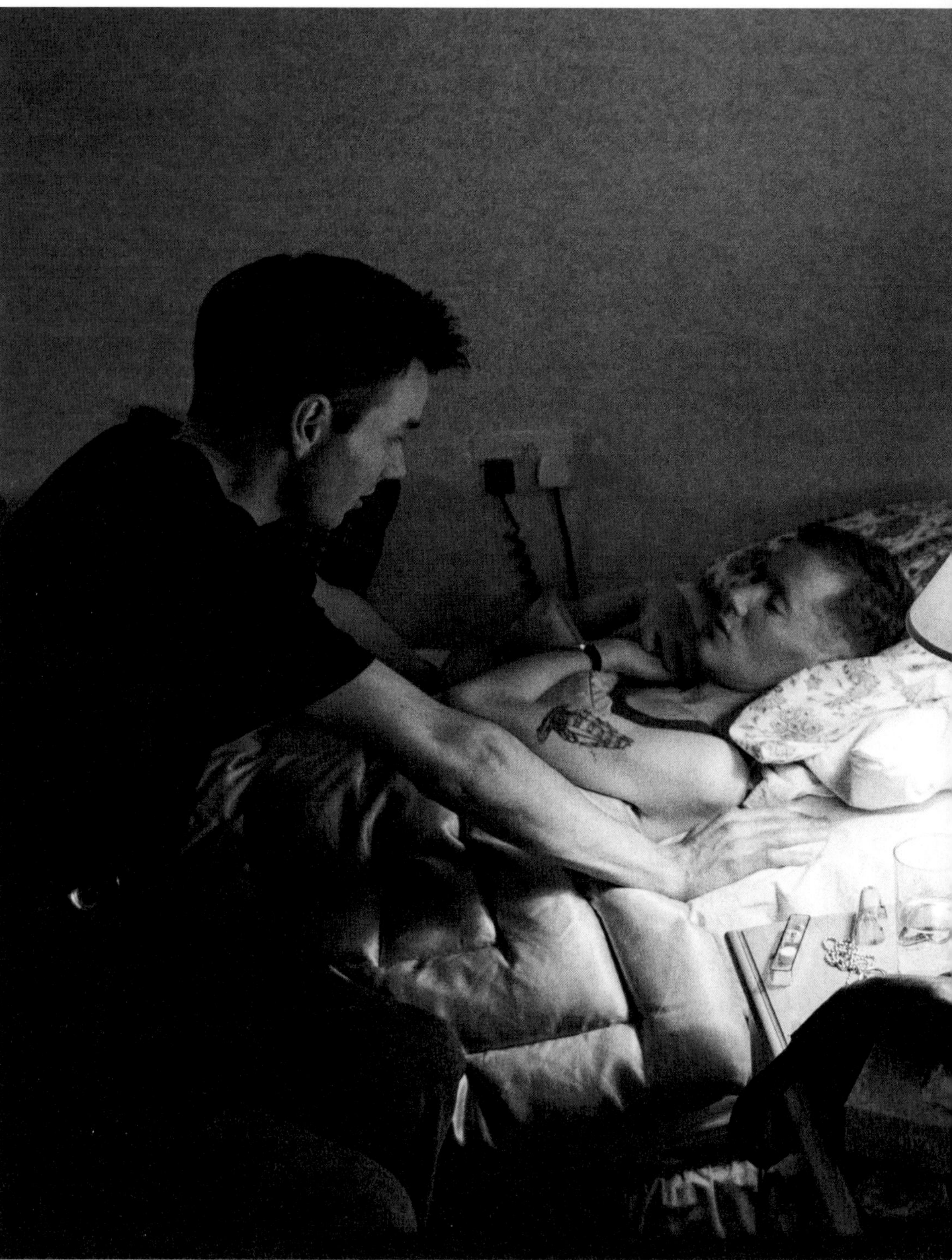

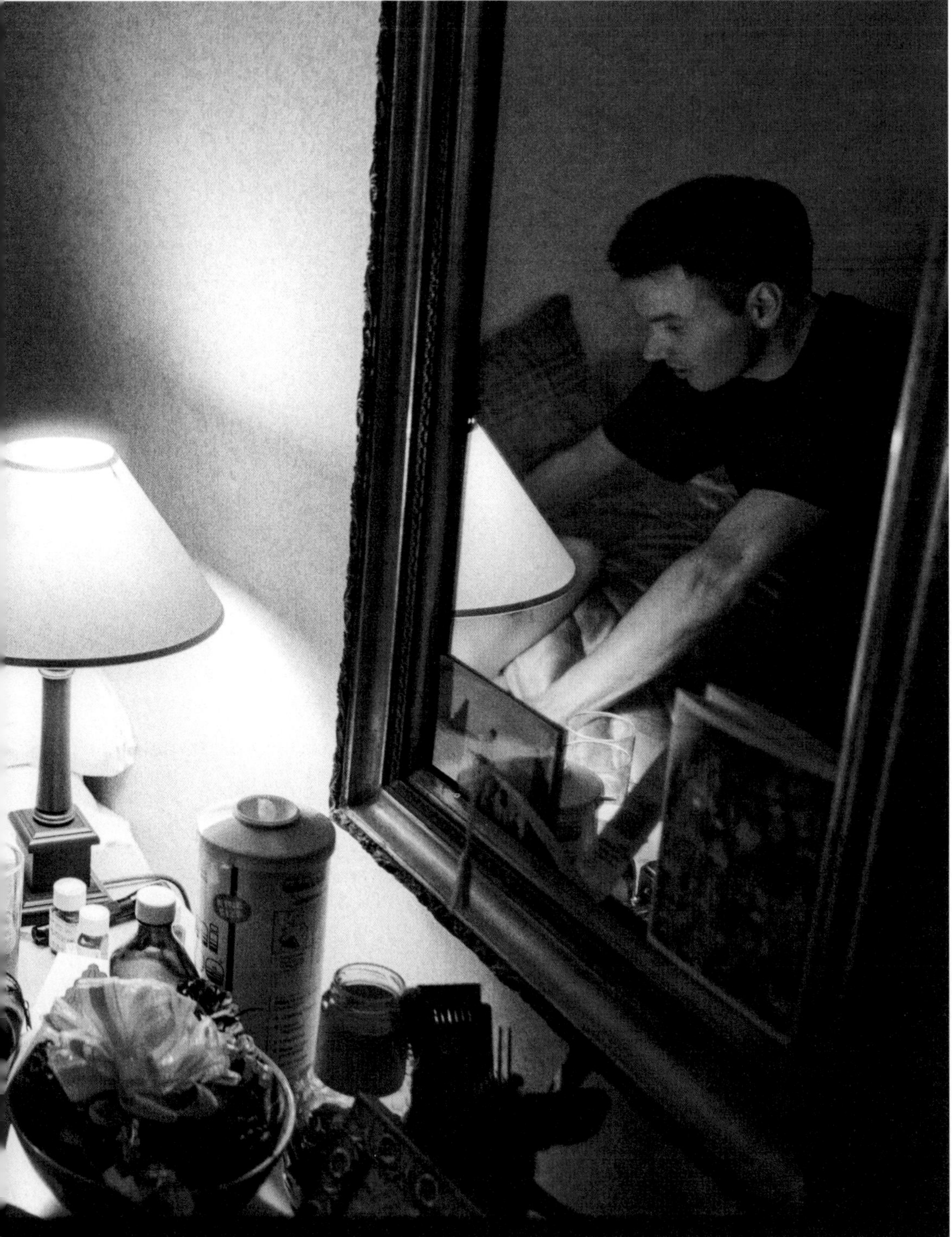

After three decades it is difficult to explain to our new generations the torment and the tenderness of those times - the vivid and painful drama in the lives of gay men and those who loved them in this terrible time as the HIV/AIDS epidemic raged through the community.

In the midst of the pain, the fear and the aching loss, were so many stories of kindness, resilience and so many creative responses. This was the central purpose of the long and complex project Positive Lives, a partnership between Terrence Higgins Trust and Network photographers which sought to tell the story of the people affected by the HIV/AIDS pandemic. It originated in a first UK exhibition and book and subsequently became a worldwide portrait of the realities of the impact and response to HIV/AIDS. Positive Lives was seen by many millions of people in so many countries and in so many different places from the UN in New York to refugee camps in Africa in a myriad of contexts used by campaigners and HIV organisations to combat stigma and increase understanding of the impact on people of this new and frightening disease which raced around the world destroying lives, hopes and dreams.

Gideon Mendel's intimate and tender portrayal of life on the ward was such an important story for Positive Lives. With his determination, sensitivity and commitment Gideon won the trust of staff and patients and was able to tell their story with such sensitivity and dignity, he showed so delicately the way these patients had transformed the constraints of hospital life - so the ward could truly serve the needs of the gay community, the hardest hit in these terrible times

Amidst all this tragedy there were also happier stories, the love and trust of those who cared for those affected, the dedication and compassion of the staff, the courage and resilience of the patients and also another story of love - for this is where Gideon met Sarah a nurse on the ward, his beautiful image of her having restorative Shiatsu massage was used to launch Positive Lives.

Lyndall Stein, co founder
of Positive Lives and Terrence Higgins Trust
Head of Fundraising 1992 - 1995

1993, so long ago. If I think back to my time on the wards I remember two things. There was the look that people would get in their eyes when they were very ill, it said, `I'm dying, I know it and you know it and there is nothing that can be done. It was the sadness and helplessness of AIDS and everything was summed up in that death filled fear filled word.

Then there was the passion and solidarity, the fight that would shine even brighter, the long days and longer nights, the lines and the drugs and the experimental treatments. There was a commitment and drive to improve things together, it redefined the doctor-patient relationship. Not just that relationship, but others, family and friends put aside what ultimately were petty prejudices to face something which was way bigger.

Dr Ade Fakoya
Registrar in HIV and Sexual Health
at UCL / Middlesex hospitals, 1993

We knew we were struggling through momentous times, but understanding exactly what the moment was became more difficult as we drowned in the crescendo of protest that was almost the only political (and in some instances, clinical) tool available to us until the mid 1990's. So it is with tremendous pride that I look again at the narratives and messages that were so carefully sculpted by the photographers of the Network agency in the period 1991-1993 in the miserable heart of the epidemic, with such subtlety, insight and power. A quarter century later I still refer to Gideon's work on the ward, with particular reference to the image of the parents sitting either side of the bed with Michael & John. We published the image shortly after John died and the parents had a brick through their window. Pain upon pain and I immediately withdrew the image from circulation. And so it stayed for a full 30 minutes until Michael called full of fury that I had overridden John's deliberate wish that his death should not pass in vain and that these images must be seen as widely as possible. He was right of course and I talk about this decision in the context of ethical conflict in

photojournalism: sometimes the ethical way forward
is against the interests of the people in the picture
and that the prevention of pain isn't necessarily the
driving consideration. There can never be a rulebook
on ethics even though each new generation argues
the need for clarity.

At that time the narrative of "planet AIDS" was
told mainly in 80 point headlines which severely
limited information, carried little nuance and
compassion was thrown deep in the negative scale.
And yet as soon as one scratched the surface it
was hard to find anyone in UK without some
connection to the epidemic. The solitary terror of
nights alone in the hospital, the bewilderment of
parents, the courage of carers, the ripped-out-heart
pain of partners, befuddlement of educators, and
one shouldn't forget the callous glee of tabloid
journalists who created the bête noir and stuck it
daily with cruel wit and panache for over a decade.
They all had a finger on the pulse of the epidemic.
In the Positive Lives book Sir John Junor's portrait by
Steve Pyke is next to his own words: "It is said that
by shaking hands with patients in an AIDS ward,
Princess Diana showed that that the disease need
not make them into social outcasts. But since each
had only his homosexual promiscuity to blame for the
disease, isn't that exactly what they should be?"

Once again I feel the anger that fuelled those
relentless protests. I fear that the solution is not as
simple as remembering; many of us remember the
worst of the epidemic and contemporary records
abound, as they do for so many humanitarian crises.
Memory is not at issue. Rather it is our own psychology that will cause this and other catastrophes
to repeat, and against which we must maintain
permanent personal vigilance. Who can I help today?

For those that made it to 2017 I have an
embrace, and for the many who didn't, I have
gratitude for what they taught me about fighting
the odds, and too many tears. I would also like to
thank Robert Grieve who gave us the brilliant title
'Positive Lives' and who died in 2011 without the
recognition he deserved for branding this huge and
complex project so succinctly.

**Stephen Mayes, co founder of Positive Lives
and former head of Network agency**

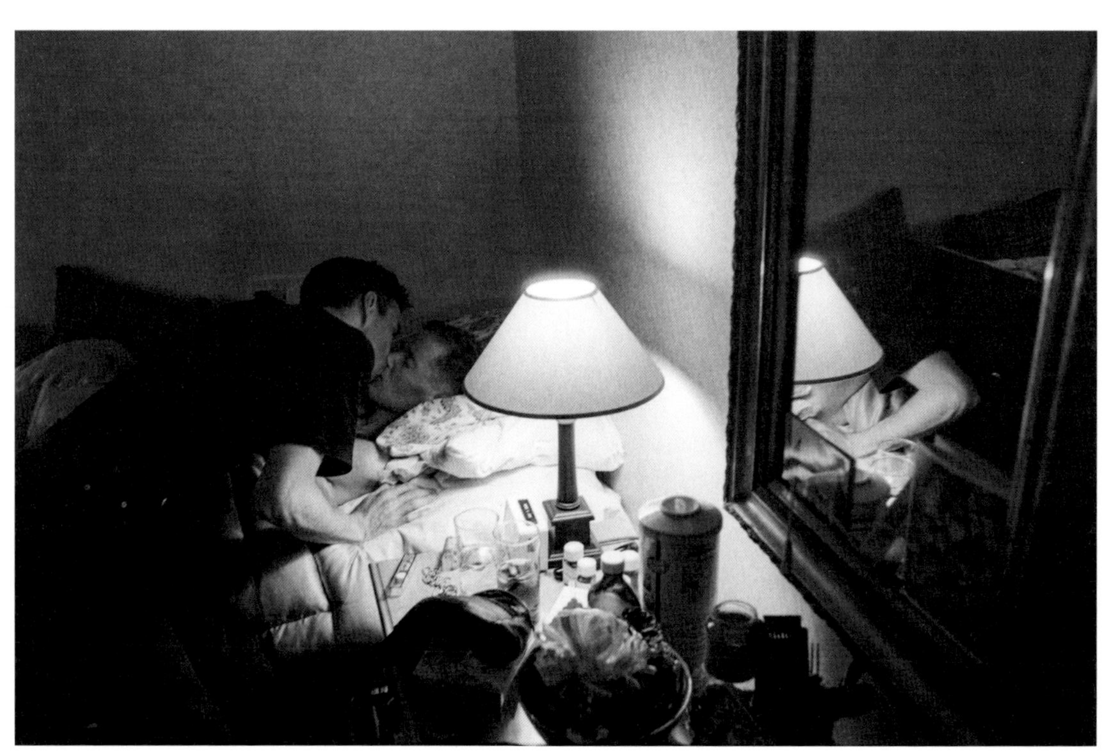

When to the sessions of sweet silent thought
I summon up remembrance of things past,
I sigh the lack of many a thing I sought,
And with old woes new wail my dear time's waste:
Then can I drown an eye, unus'd to flow,
For precious friends hid in death's dateless night,
And weep afresh love's long since cancell'd woe,
And moan the expense of many a vanish'd sight:
Then can I grieve at grievances foregone,
And heavily from woe to woe tell o'er
The sad account of fore-bemoaned moan,
Which I new pay as if not paid before.
But if the while I think on thee, dear friend,
All losses are restor'd and sorrows end.

Shakespeare, Sonnet 30

**Chosen by Carlos Silva de Santa Anna,
for his partner Geoge Leslie Boyd Leivers
who died on the ward 13th August 1993.**

Thank you to The Fitzrovia Chapel, the only remaining building of The Middlesex Hospital, for presenting two exhibitions of The Ward and supporting the second edition of this book and to Hannah Watson whose energy and resourcefulness made them both happen. Lyndall Stein and Stephen Mayes directed the ground breaking Positive Lives project in 1993, which helped bring these images into the world. Jane Bruton, sister of the Broderip ward was an inspiring figure for many who trusted me to bring my camera into her patients' lives, and has continued to be a collaborator in my ongoing work on HIV.

Most importantly we need to appreciate the amazing bravery, in the face of extreme stigma, of John, Andre, Steven and Ian - along with their partners, friends and families - for allowing my camera into such intimate moments of their lives.

Photographs © Gideon Mendel
Text © Dr Jane Anderson, Dr Denise Barulis, Jane Bruton, Robert Chevara, Dr Duncan Churchill, Julian Clary, Dr Ade Fakoya, Sarah Macauley, Stephen Mayes, Chris Mazeika, Professor Rob Miller, Angelina Namiba, Sir Nick Partridge, Chris Sandford, Lyndall Stein, Barbara Von Barsewisch, Dr Shamil Wanigaratne and Heather Wilson.

Design by Jamie Shaw

ISBN 978 - 1 - 907112 - 56 - 0

Printed in Italy by Grafiche Antiga
Second edition published in Great Britain in 2022
by Trolley Ltd
www.trolleybooks.com

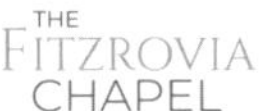